BASICS IN BURNS FOR NURSES

BASICS IN BURNS FOR NURSES

Prema Dhanraj
MS M Ch(Plastic) FACS CTBS PDFBR (USA)

Professor and Head
Department of Plastic Surgery
Christian Medical College (CMC)
Vellore, Tamil Nadu, India

Foreword

Robert L McCauley

JAYPEE

JAYPEE BROTHERS MEDICAL PUBLISHERS
The Health Sciences Publisher
New Delhi | London

Jaypee Brothers Medical Publishers (P) Ltd

Headquarters
EMCA House, 23/23-B
Ansari Road, Daryaganj
New Delhi 110 002, India
Landline: +91-11-23272143, +91-11-23272703
+91-11-23282021, +91-11-23245672
e-mail: jaypee@jaypeebrothers.com

Corporate Office
4838/24, Ansari Road, Daryaganj
New Delhi 110 002, India
Phone: +91-11-43574357
Fax: +91-11-43574314
e-mail: jaypee@jaypeebrothers.com

Overseas Office
JP Medical Ltd.
83, Victoria Street, London
SW1H 0HW (UK)
Phone: +44-20 3170 8910
e-mail: info@jpmedpub.com

EU GPSR Authorised Representative
Logos Europe, 9 rue Nicolas Poussin
17000, La Rochelle, France
Phone: +33 (0) 6 67 93 73 78
e-mail: contact@logoseurope.eu

Website: www.jaypeebrothers.com
Website: www.jaypeedigital.com

Inquiries for bulk sales may be solicited at: jaypee@jaypeebrothers.com

Basics in Burns for Nurses

First Edition: 2011, **Reprint: 2025**

ISBN: 978-93-5025-068-6

Printed in India

To

My Parents
Late Mr Dhanraj
and
Late Mrs Rosey Dhanraj

FOREWORD

The author, Prema Dhanraj, has written a comprehensive text for care of burn patients from the perspective of nurses.

First and foremost in the mind of this basics are the responsibilities of the nursing team. The book is well organized into key sections. The first section includes an introduction to burns, which outlines the pathophysiology of burns, as well as the role of nursing in the management of these devastating injuries. Section two of the book begins with acute burn care management. This includes fluid resuscitation to maintain fluid balance in these very difficult patients. Other issues addressed include pain management, tissue substitutes, the use of skin grafts and outpatient care. All of these issues are developed from the nurse's perspective. Early and late complications of burn injuries are also addressed. The book ends with sections on reconstruction and rehabilitation of the burn patient. Again here we have a comprehensive guide with the focus on nursing care and other nursing issues.

The author should be commended on this very comprehensive work. It is clear that not only seasoned nurses will benefit from this basics but also nursing students, medical students, and other health care professionals who are dedicated to the difficult task of taking care of burn patients. Indeed, the information contained in this manual for nurses, is comprehensive and clear. This body of work certainly is a valuable addition to our current literature dedicated to the care of burn patients.

Robert L McCauley MD FACS
Professor and Chief
of Plastic and Reconstructive Surgery
University of Texas Medical Branch
Shriners Hospital for Children
Galveston, Texas USA

PREFACE

The title *Basics in Burns for Nurses* was in response to a search for a pocket-sized concise reference book on burns for nurses, medical students, private practitioners and to all those who are involved in the care of a burn patients.

The goal of this manual is to present the entire scope of burns in a simple, easy-to-read format.

I hope that the reader will find this book useful in day-to-day management of burns.

Prema Dhanraj

Contents

Section One : Introduction to Burns

Section Two : Acute Care

Section Three : Complications: Early and Late

Section Four : Reconstruction

Section Five : Rehabilitation

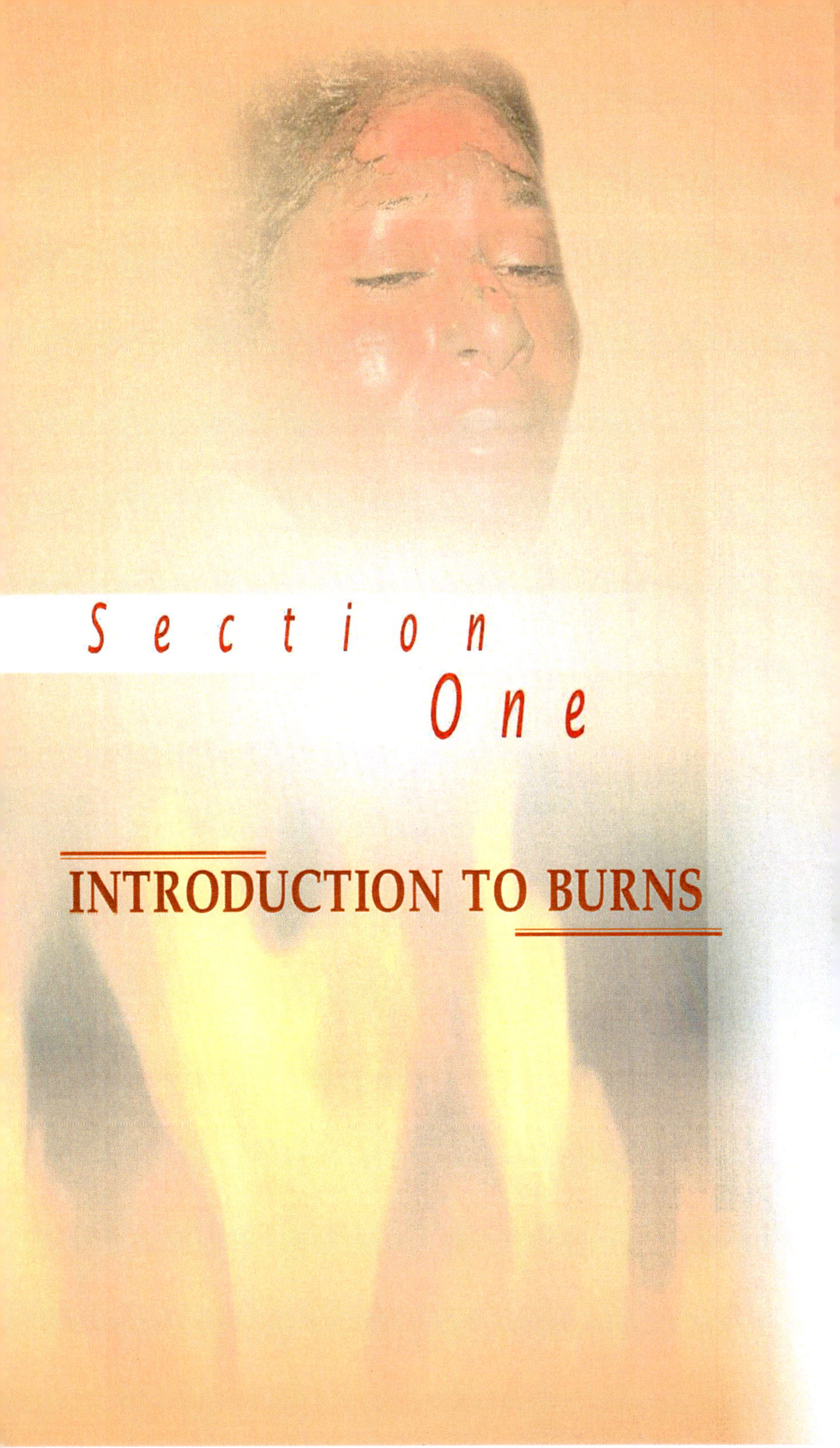

Section One

INTRODUCTION TO BURNS

Chapter 1 INTRODUCTION

Burns occur universally. Incidence is on the increase with the complexities of modern living and industrialization. Although burns are a major problem in India it has not received the attention it deserves. Probably due to the cost of hospitalization and care which imposes a severe burden on the limited resources. Since most of the burns occur either at home or at work place it is important for every one to know the first aid management of burns.

India is a vast land with huge population of over a billion, of which 80% live in rural areas where modern medical facilities are not available. Over 7 million burn injuries occur every year, may be even higher considering a high rate of illiteracy, poverty, poor standards of safety at home and at work place, marital problems, floor level cooking, defective appliances and traditional loose garments.

Burn injuries are a major challenge to most hospital medical and nursing staff. The physiologic response to injury is complex and the cost of treatment is exorbitant.

The treatment is painstaking, expensive and can still lead to deformity, disfigurement, disability, prolonged rehabilitation, loss of income, job and an enormous financial burden to families.

Specialized burn centers available in this country are too few for the magnitude of the problem, as a result of which majority of patients are treated by surgeons in the peripheral districts with meager resources.

The traditional Doctor – Nurse is grossly inadequate to provide the comprehensive care required by burn patients. Burn specialists and trained nurses are in short supply. Further the problem is compounded by lack of proper medical facilities for specialized treatment. Lack of financial resources, lack of burn education, lack of skin bank, non availability of blood for transfusion is all the limiting factors. The biggest misfortune is the social stigma attached to the burn deformities, which produces a grim scenario for the burn victims. Illiteracy and poverty continue to create hurdles in burn prevention strategy. Education on prevention of burns is still inadequate. First aid in burns is also quite primitive due to lack of education.

Although rapid progress has been made in the care of the burned patient over the past few decades.

In the early 1950's – Importance of fluid resuscitation and the impact of delay in resuscitation on burn mortality was better understood.

In the late 1960's – New topical antimicrobial agents became available

In the 1980's – a. Importance was given to early excision and closure of the burn wound

– b. Better understanding of the pathophysiology of the burn injury

– c. Concept of a burn team

Most of the progress has not reached the rural India.

Considering that the burn team is a multidisciplinary team and all play a great part in the care of the burn victim, burn nursing presents a challenge to a nurse, because their contribution is worthwhile. Nurses form the core team in "Hands on care" and need to keep an open mind and be aware of newer developments. A nurse is the most important link between the team members. A lot of responsibility rests on her information as the clinician plans the treatment strategy based on her observation. Hence it is extremely helpful to have a nurse with good knowledge of burn nursing as she can guide, monitor and analyze the patient's condition so that the best care can be provided.

The magnitude of severe burn injury presents a difficult nursing problem as they have to cope with high physical demand of high dependency patients, thus the role of nurse becomes highly stressful. It is therefore important to rotate them now and then with in the general plastic surgery ward to reduce the "**Burn out syndrome**".

Chapter 2

NURSING

2.1 NURSING PRINCIPLES

- Observation on admission
- Resuscitation
  - Weight of the patient
  - Estimation of burn injury
  - Collection of blood
  - Fluid calculation and replacement
  - Insert urinary catheter
  - Monitor vital signs
  - Insert nasogastric tube
- Care of the burn wound
  - Immediate care
  - Planned care
  - Splinting of extremities
  - Physiotherapy
  - Grafting
- Nursing care
  - Specific nursing care
  - General nursing care
- Nutrition and Feeding
  - Daily nutritional requirement
  - Additional requirements for burns
- Emotional and social support
  - Maintain proper conversation and comm- unication with the patient
  - Involve relatives, near and dear ones, colleagues and acquaintances
  - Periodic visit of a completely cured and rehabilitated burn patient can inspire and encourage rehabilitation

• Complications	– Immediate during first 48-72 hours
	– Delayed
• Rehabilitation	– Encourage self adaptation
	– Frequent visits by senior colleagues
• Education	– prevention of burns
	– Education of relatives during treatment, convalescence
	– Education of patients to adapt and learn to accept

- The ultimate aim of a nurse is to make the patient to go back to the place where he belongs.

Chapter

3 ROLE OF A NURSE IN THE MANAGEMENT OF BURNS

3.1 IMMEDIATE

- Estimate burn injury
- Weigh the patient/approximate weight calculated from height and age
- Set the trolley for intravenous line/urinary catheterization and nasogastric tube insertion
- Intravenous fluids like normal saline/dextrose saline
- Blood tubes for collection of blood for investigation.

3.2 CARE OF THE PATIENT

- Monitor vital signs
- Observe level of consciousness
- Elevate head end and extremities
- Remove bangles and rings to avoid constriction and hand it over to relatives.

3.3 INVESTIGATION

Blood samples should be sent to lab and results collected for hemoglobin, electrolytes, RBS, creatinine, total protein and albumin.

3.4 CARE OF THE BURN WOUND

- Assess the type of burn and plan for appropriate dressing
- Splint the areas in the position of function.

3.5 NUTRITION

On the first day insert nasogastric tube and start simple nutrients like butter milk (prepare one cup of curd and three cups of water). This simple nutrient keeps the normal bowel movement . Give 50 ml of buttermilk hourly and aspirate every 4th hourly to check retention of fluid.

Calculate the calorie requirement using Curreri formula. Give half strength of this formula at 50 ml/hour and continue to aspirate every 4th hour for retention of fluid. On the third day full strength formula is given orally. If the patient is unable to take the whole requirement orally then supplement food should be given in the form of a drip continuously so as to avoid diarrhea and vomiting.

3.6 INSERT INDWELLING CATHETER

Hourly urine output should be measured 0.5 – 1 ml/kg/hour of urine should be maintained at all times. This is the best guideline.

3.7 SYSTEMIC ANTIBIOTIC

Injection crystalline penicillin 10 L every 6th hourly administered after test dose.

3.8 EMOTIONAL SUPPORT

Be kind to the patient and relatives. Communicate with the patient and be supportive. Give a patient hearing to the problems.

3.9 POSITION

Make the patient comfortable. Talk to the relatives and brief them about the condition of the patient and allow them to see the patient.

3.10 LEGAL ISSUES

- Consider all burn cases as a medicolegal case (MLC)
- Check for incident report and inform the hospital
- The hospital will in turn inform the police
- Obtain the address and tele phone number of the relatives.

Thus the role of a nurse is to assess, plan, implement and evaluate the care of the burn patient. Burn nurses also form an important link between all the disciplines providing care to the burn patient. The burn nurses co-ordinate and provide quality care to burn patients throughout their treatment phase.

Specific Attention to Area's Affected by Burns

1. **Face:** Clean with saline and apply non adherent paraffin gauze with neosporin ointment. This dressing is removed gently every day and a fresh one applied without injuring the new epithelium.
2. **Eyes:** Irrigate the eyes with saline, apply eyedrops and get an ophthalmologist to evaluate the status of the eye.
3. **Nose:** Clean the nose with moist/wet gauze pieces /swab sticks, lubricate the nostrils to prevent crusting. If the nostril size is becoming smaller use red rubber tube lubricated and placed in the nostril to prevent stenosis.
4. **Mouth :** Give mouth care after every feed , apply liquid paraffin to the lips to prevent drying and crusting.
5. **Neck:** Avoid pillow, give a shoulder pillow to extend the neck, use a soft sponge roll as cervical collar (use a 6" bandage wrapped in the big gauze for tie over).
6. **Axilla:** Clean the axilla often to prevent infection . Place a soft sponge roll and abduct the shoulder.
7. **Hand**: Hands should be cleaned under water to make it comfortable for the patient once the dressing is removed under water, hydrotherapy should be encouraged. Place a ball to play in the water. Ask the patient to squeeze the ball and move all the fingers. Importance should be given to the web spaces while dressing, a moist gauze piece should be kept between each web space to prevent maceration and contracture.
8. **Feet:** Care is taken to dress the wound and the web spaces. Position the feet by splinting and elevating.
9. **Extremities:** Once the dressing is done use splints to keep them in extension. Elevation of the limbs by either using a pillow or keeping BB splint.

Discipline in Burn Unit

As a Nurse

- Dress as per the code maintaining the discipline
- Clean and well pressed/ironed uniform
- Hair tucked in properly

- Keep finger nails short
- Be pleasant.

Be Punctual

- In reporting on duty
- Maintaining fluid balance documents
- Document vital signs and any change in vital signs.

Prompt Reporting

- Change in the level of consciousness
- Change in patients behavior
- Quantity difference in urinary output
- Vomiting
- Diarrhea
- Change in lab investigation.

Chapter 4

ANATOMY AND PHYSIOLOGY OF SKIN

Structure

Skin is composed of two layers, the epidermis and the dermis. The epidermis is the outer layer and the dermis is the inner layer (Fig. 4.1).

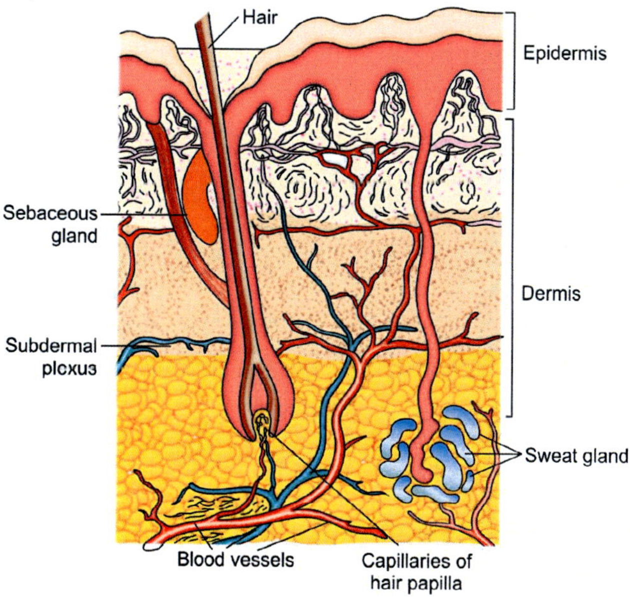

Fig. 4.1: Anatomy of skin

Epidermis

It is composed of five layers from superficial to deep

- Stratum corneum
- Stratum lucidum

- Stratum granulosum
- Stratum spinosum
- Stratum germinative (basal layer).

Epidermis consists of stratified squamous epithelium. The deepest layer consists of tall columar cells and flatten as they reach the surface.

Dermis

Dermis has two layers –Papillary and reticular layer. Dermis is formed of fibrous connective tissue. Various epidermal structures like sweat glands, sebaceous glands and hair follicle invade the dermis.

Function of Skin

Skin is the largest organ in the body and acts as a first line of defense.

- Prevents loss of body fluids, electrolytes and proteins
- Controls body temperature, allows rapid cooling and vasodilatation of dermal vessels
- Functions as excretory and sensory organs and interprets pain, touch, hot and cold
- It protects from weather, harmful environment and radiation
- It prevents entry of microorganisms and protects against infection
- It helps in production of vitamin D.

Chapter 5

TYPES OF BURNS

Flame Burns

A. Definition: Burns means thermal injury. It results in coagulative alteration of proteins due to wide range of temperatures, ranging from the lowest—that is frostbite to the highest—that is electrical injury. Thus both extremes of heat and cold can cause burn injury.

B. Epidemiology

- Seven million sustain burns
- Three million die/year
- 75 % of burns occur at home
- 80 % involve women and children.

C. Etiology

- Illiteracy
- Poor living condition
- Marital problems
- Floor level cooking
- Traditional loose garments
- Defective appliances.

D. Important changes in treatment

- Cool the burn surface with water (Fig. 5.1).
- To use crystalloids for volume resuscitation
- Isolated rooms with intensive care facilities
- Early enteral nutrition
- Better management of sepsis
- Advanced wound management.

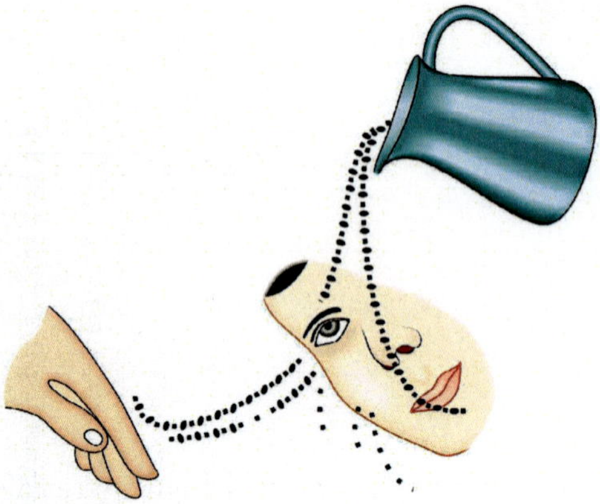

Fig. 5.1: Cool the burn surface with water

E. First Aid Management

- Water
  - To put off the fire (Fig. 5.2)
  - To cool the burn surface
  - To limit the initial and progressive injury
  - Start IV Fluids or give sips of water with a pinch of salt
  - Cover with a clean sheet
  - Transport to a nearest hospital.

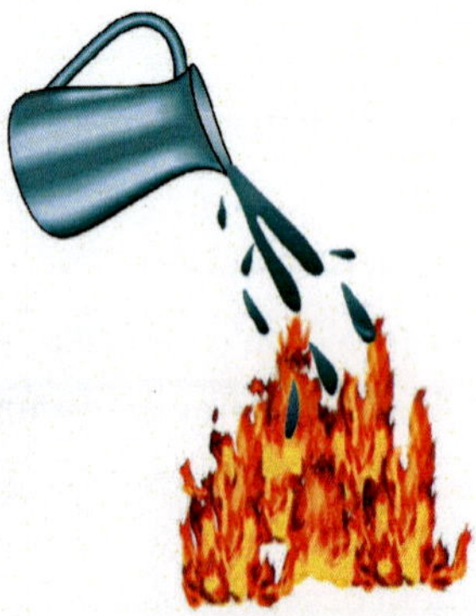

Fig. 5.2: Pour water to put off fire

F. Requirment for fluid calculation

- Weight of patient
- Percentage of burns –Rule of Nines
- Time of burns

G. Causes of burns

a. Thermal or flame burns occur due to dry heat. Seventy five percent of burns occur at home and are preventable (Fig. 5.3).

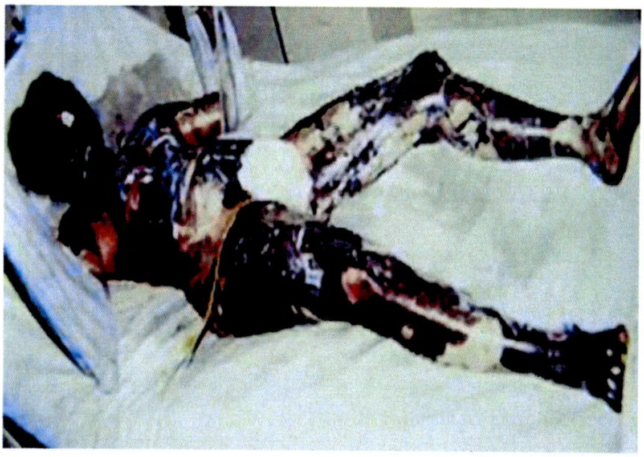

Fig. 5.3: Flame burns

b. Scald burns are due to hot liquids, mostly in children while pulling down or knocking hot liquids onto themselves (Fig. 5.4).

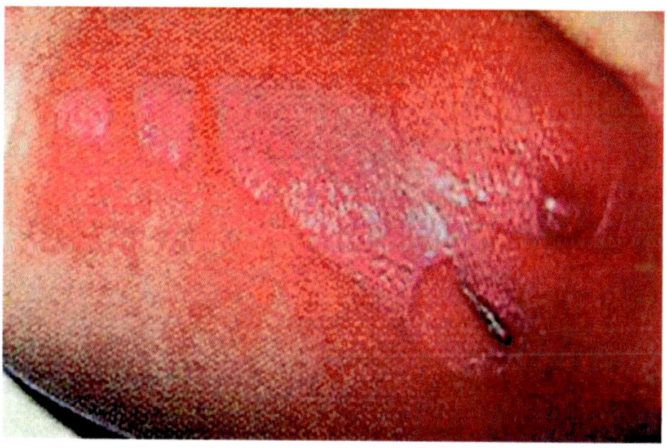

Fig. 5.4: Scald burns

c. Chemical burns are caused by strong acids and alkali. It causes tissue damage by denaturation of the cell protein. Chemical burns are unique because there is continuous tissue damage. It usually occurs at home where the acid is stored for use of cleaning toilets. Homicidal burns are very common in India due to local hooligans who throw acid on young female's face when they reject advances. Immediate removal of clothes and continuous irrigation for at least 30 minutes with water is the most effective measure of first aid management (Figs 5.5 and 5.6).

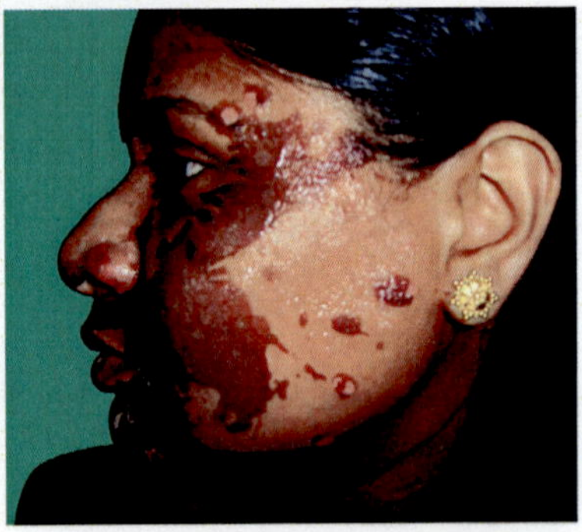

Fig. 5.5: Alkalie burns of face

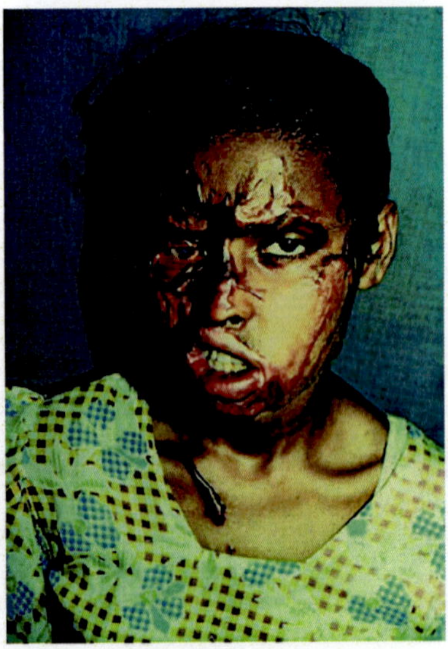

Fig. 5.6: Acid burns

d. Electrical burns can be flash, arc or contact. The flash may ignite clothes and hence burns may be superficial. In contact burns the person comes in contact with live wires. The current enters the body through nerves and vessels and exits at another site (Figs 5.7 and 5.8).

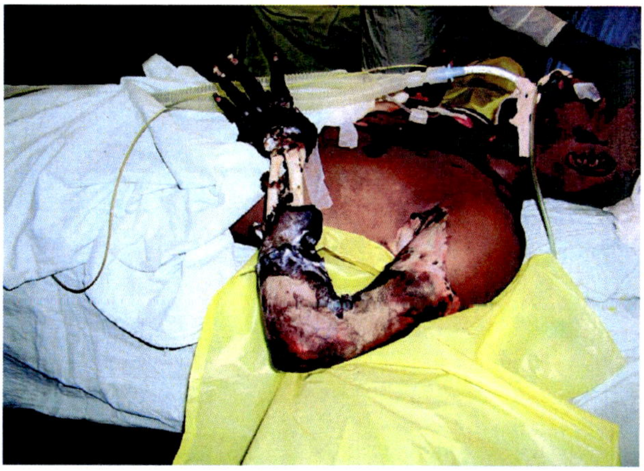

Fig. 5.7: Electrical burns with exposed bones

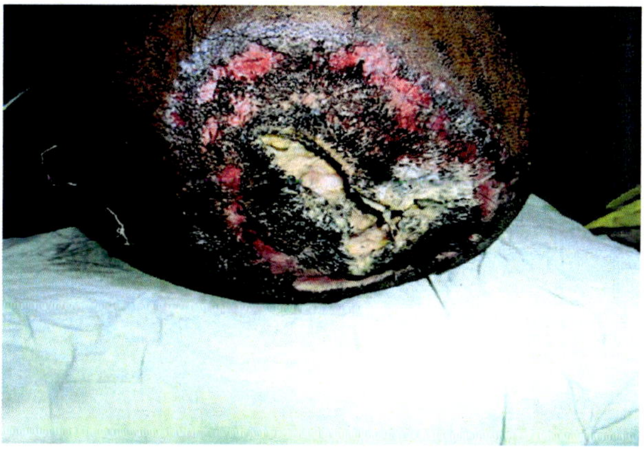

Fig. 5.8: Contact burns with charred skin

H. Assessment of burn injury

a. **Estimating burn size:** For children under 12 years of age **Lund and Browder's** formula chart is used to estimate the total body surface area burn involved (Fig. 5.9).

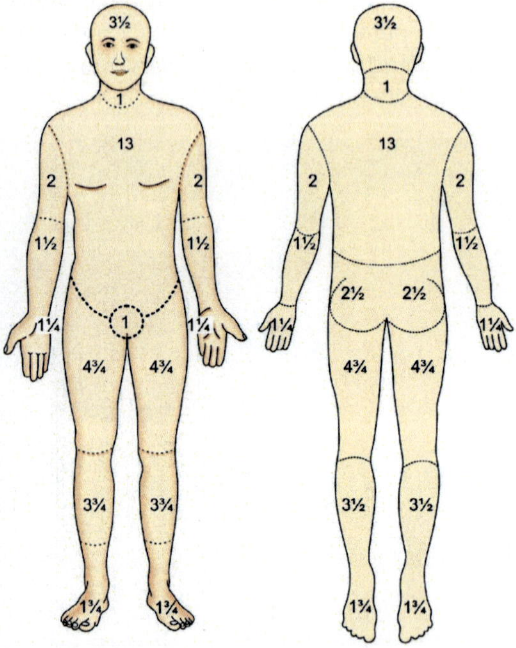

Fig. 5.9: Lund and Browder formula chart

For adults, Wallace's **"Rule of Nines"** is commonly used. According to this head and neck constitute 9% of TBSA, each upper extremity is 9%, each lower extremity is 18% and anterior and posterior trunk are 18% each, and 1% for the genitalia (Fig. 5.10).

For all age groups palmar surface of the patient's hand represents 1% of TBSA burns.

b. **Estimating burn depth:** The depth of burn determines the type of healing, besides being a prognostic factor. Burn wounds are classified according to **Boyer** into three degrees (Fig. 5.11)

First-degree burns is characterized by epidermal involvement, erythema and edema, typical example is a sunburn or touch of a hot iron. This type of burn heals spontaneously in 7 days (Fig. 5.12).

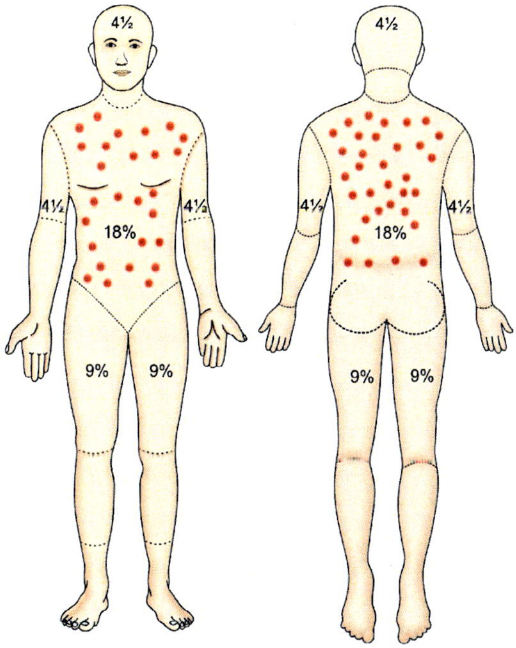

Fig. 5.10: Rule of nines

Second-degree burns are divided into superficial and deep depending upon the involvement of the dermal stru

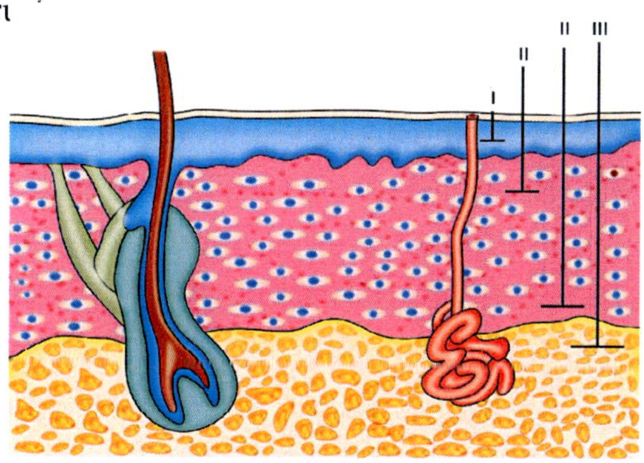

Fig. 5.11: Three degrees of burns

Second degree superficial burns involve the whole of epidermis and a small part of the dermis. Clinically blisters and blebs are seen. It blanches on pressure. The wound looks pink in color. It is also painful. The wound heals spontaneously in 7-14 days by regeneration of epithelial cells that is, hair follicles, sweat glands and sebaceous glands. Wound healing can be hastened by using skin substitutes (Figs 5.13 to 5.20).

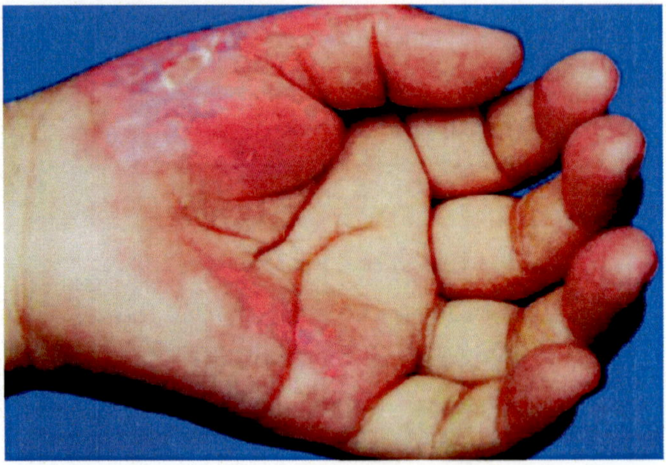

Fig. 5.12: First degree burns

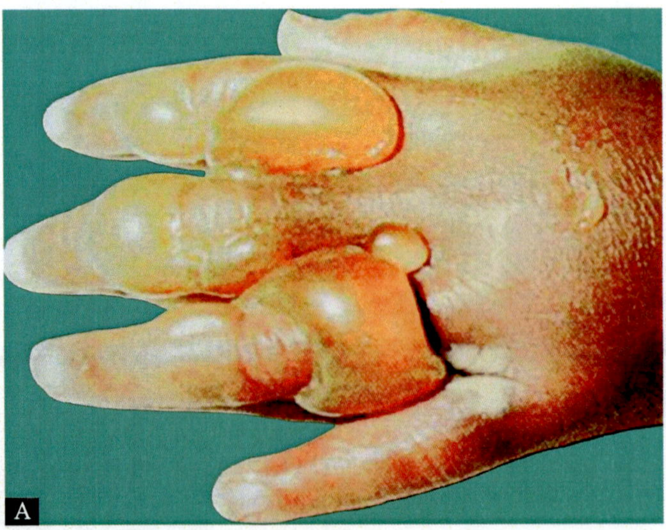

A

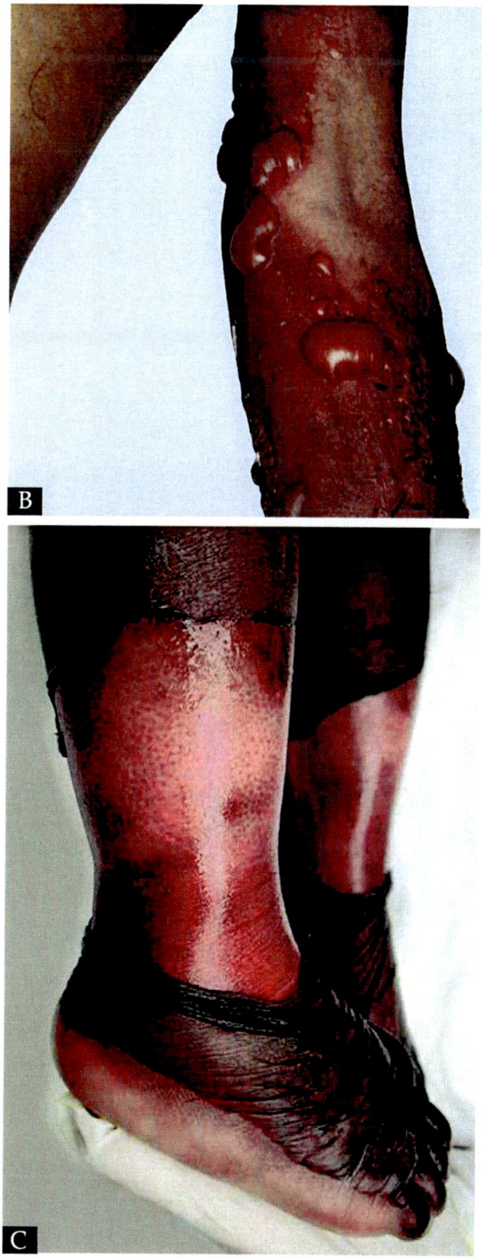

Figs 5.13 A to C: Second degree superficial burn with blisters

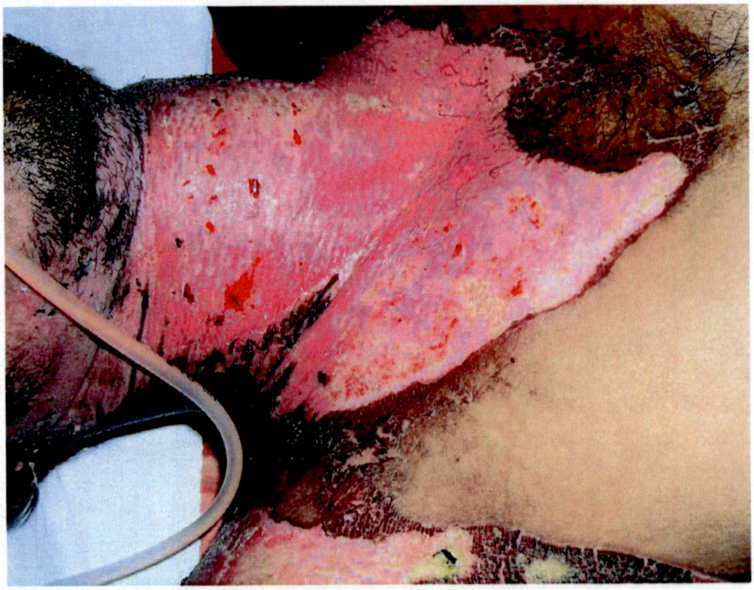

Fig. 5.14: Second degree superficial burn healed spontaneously

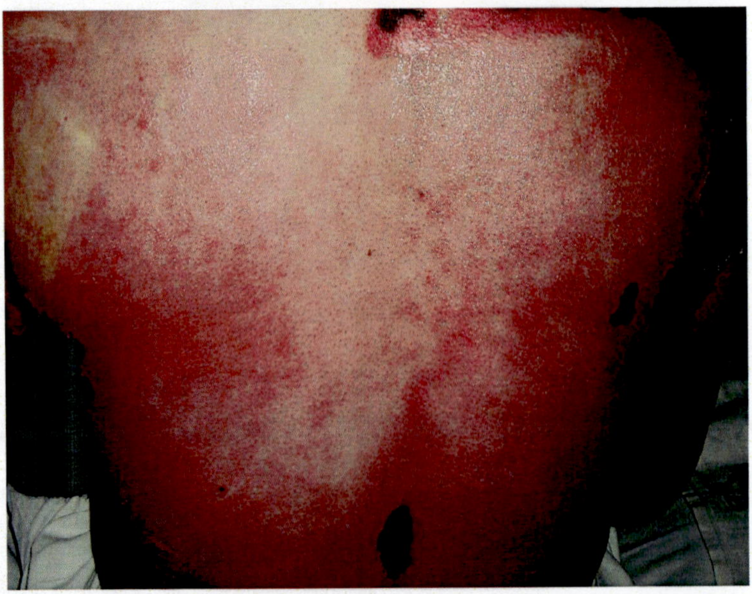

Fig. 5.15: Deep second degree burns

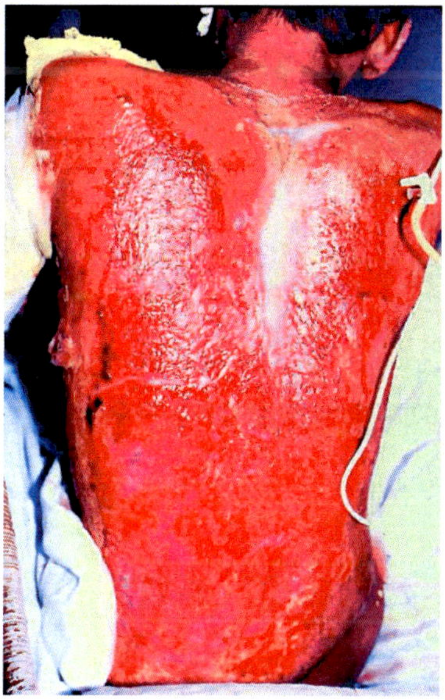

Fig. 5.16: Amnion for back

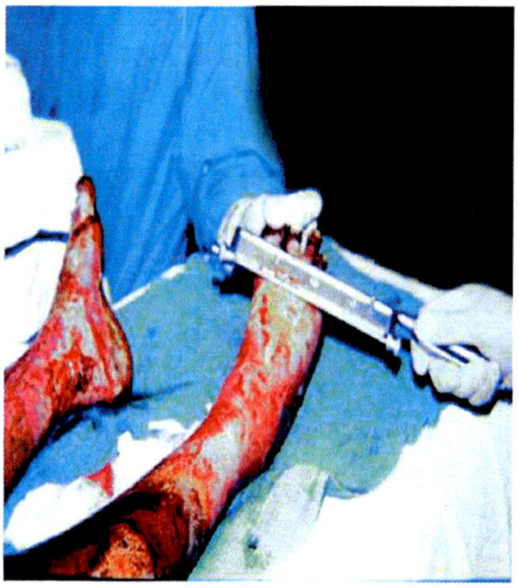

Fig. 5.17: Second degree deep—tangential excision

Second-degree deep burns involve the whole of epidermis and varying depths of dermis. It has pink white dry appearance and less painful. Epithelialization occurs more slowly due to few epithelial structures present in the dermis. If infection sets in, this type of burns gets easily converted to third degree burns (Figs 5.21 to 5.27).

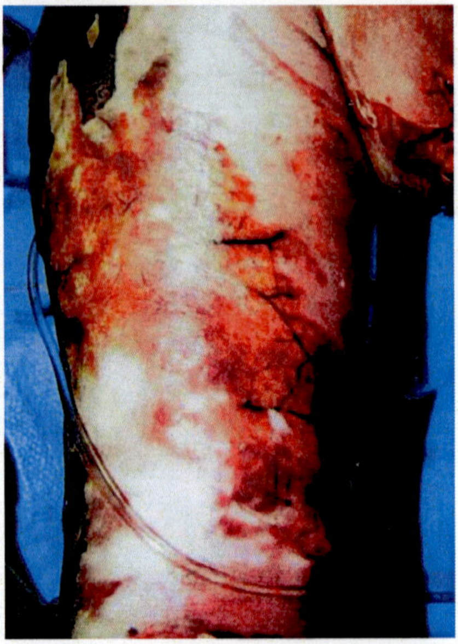

Fig. 5.18: Third degree burns with coagulated veins

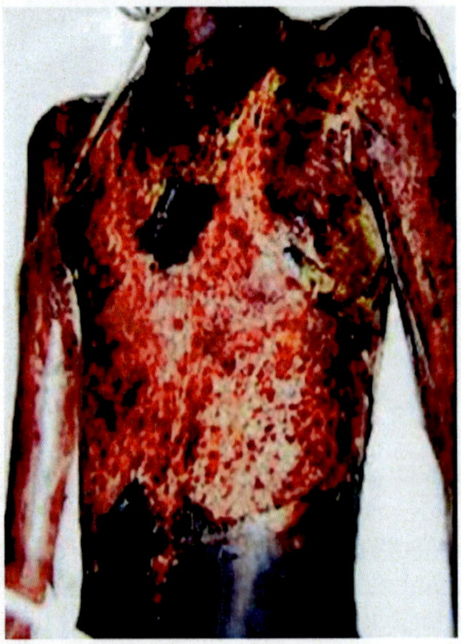

Fig. 5.19: Third degree burns with thick eschar

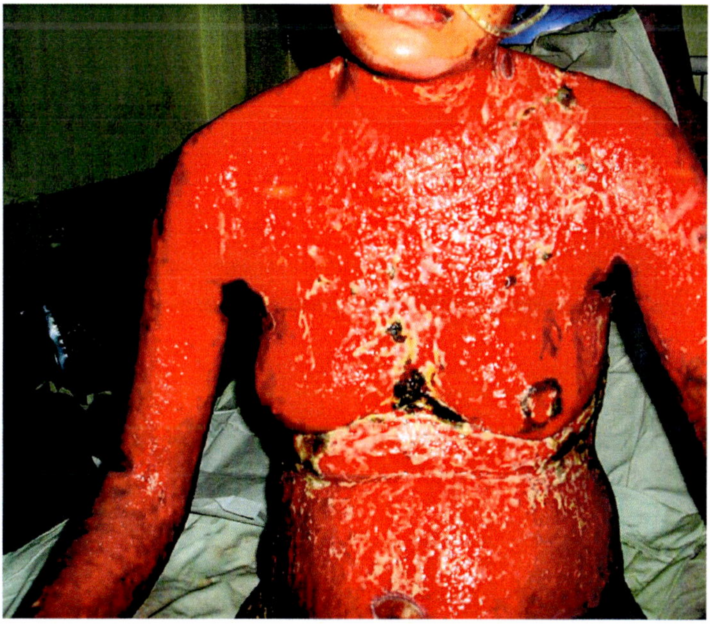

Fig. 5.20: Third degree burns after complete eschar removal

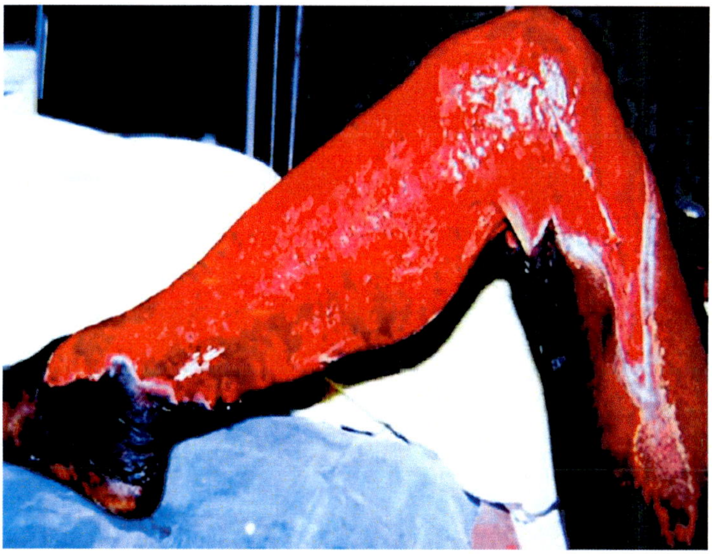

Fig. 5.21: Third degree burns with good granulation tissue ready for grafting

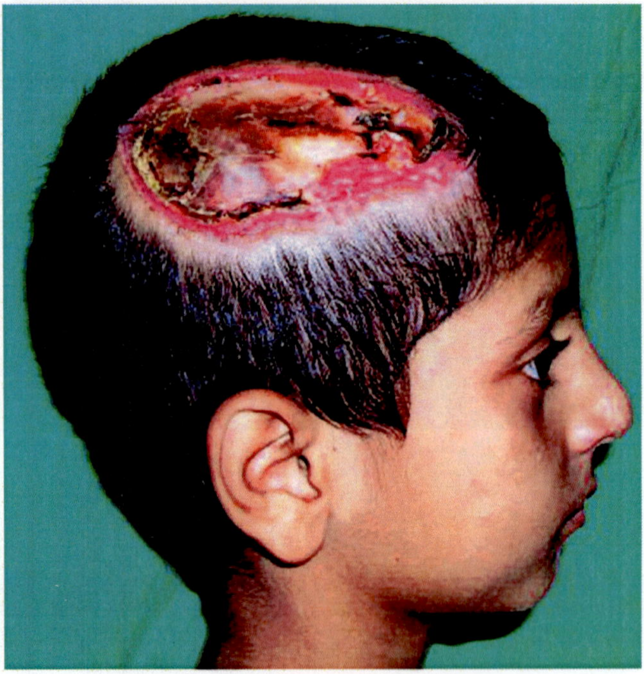

Fig. 5.22: Contact burns with necrosed bone

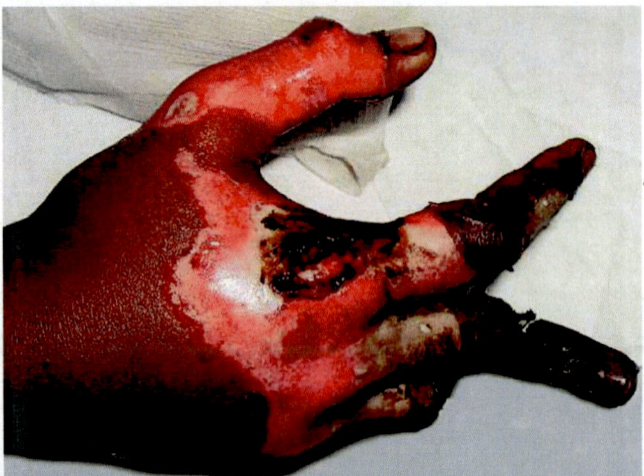

Fig. 5.23: Electrical burns of hand with charred finger

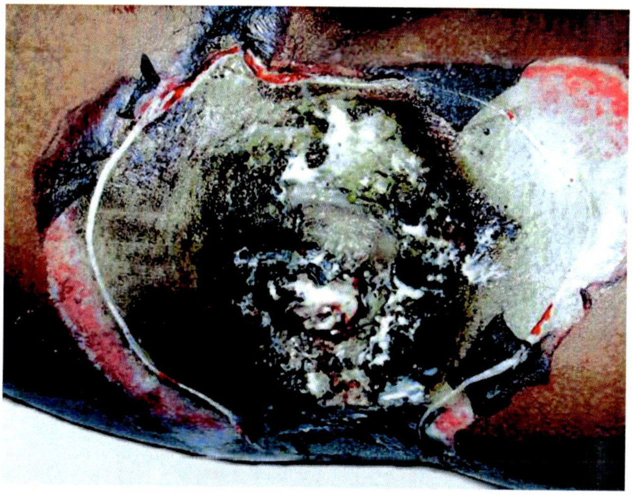

Fig. 5.24: Electrical burns of thigh with exposed bone

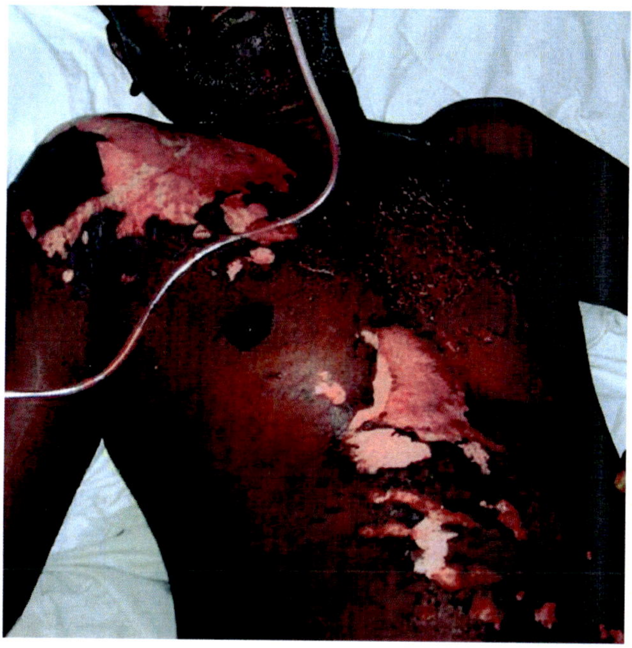

Fig. 5.25: Electrical flash burn

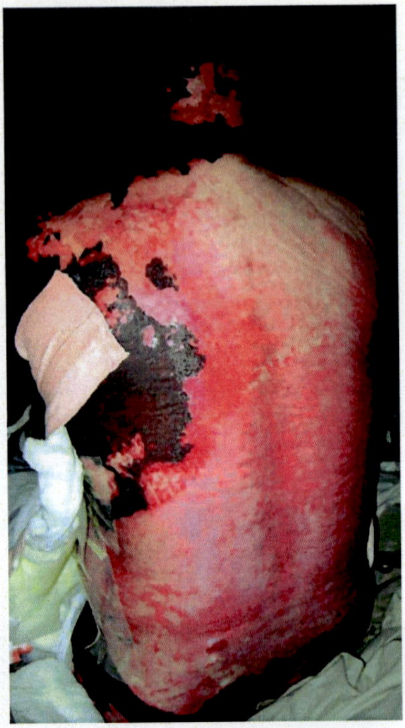

Fig. 5.26: Electrical flash burn back

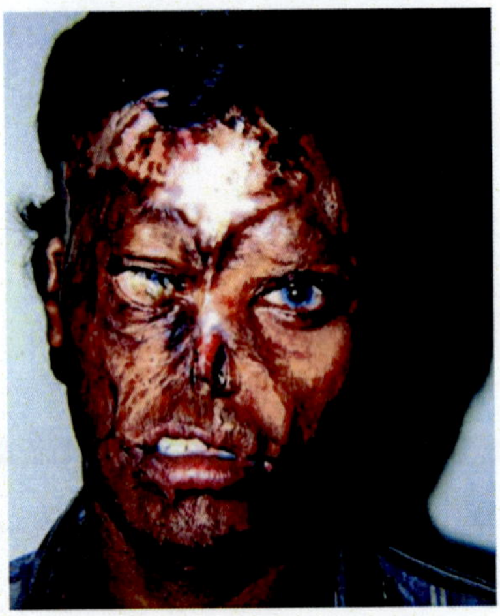

Fig. 5.27: Acid burns

Third degree burns involves the whole of epidermis, the whole of dermis and different depths of subcutaneous tissue. It appears white, brown or black. The surface is dry and leathery. Coagulated veins are seen on the surface pain is characteristically absent. Collagen, a protein present in the dermis turns white on burning, charring of this collagen results in black color. This type of burns will not heal spontaneously and treatment is by excision and grafting.

Summary

Burn depth	Clinical features	Treatment
First degree burns Typical exmple is a sun burn/touch of a hot iron box	Epidermal involvement Erythema–red color Edema	- Apply topical ointments like Neosporin - Heals in 7 days
Second degree superficial involves epidermis and a small part of dermis	Blister, blebs and bullae Pink in color (subdermal plexus seen through) painful moist blanches with pressure	- Apply non adherent dressings OR - Synthetic skin substitutes/ amnion/healicoll - Heals spontaneously in 7-14 days due to re epithe lialization from the hair follicle, sweat glands and seba ceous glands
Second degree deep Involves epidermis and most of dermis	Pink white appearance Blistering not seen Dry appearance Ischemic at the center and hyperemic at the periphery does not blanch with pressure	- Early tangential excision and grafting is the best option - If the wound does not heal spontaneously in 3 weeks - surgical excision and grafting.
Third degree burns Involves epidermis Dermis and varying depths of subcutaneous tissue	- Appears dry and depressed - Color can be white brown or black (white because the collagen being a protein turns white on heating) - Skin feels leathery - Coagulated veins are seen through - Pain absent	Tangential excision and grafting (does not heal spontaneously as all the epidermal structures like hair follicle, sweat glands and sebaceous glands are destroyed)

Electrical Burns

Electrical burns are complex injuries and may affect multiple organs. Most tissue damage is caused by heat generated by current flow leading to progressive loss of viable tissue due to delayed thrombosis of microvasculature. Prevention and treatment are important.

Classification

- Low voltage <1000 volts causes local tissue necrosis.
- High voltage >1000 voltage causes deep muscle injury and fractures.
- Ultra high voltage seen in lightening injury, blast injury resulting in cardiac arrest.

Type of Injury

It damages tissues in three ways —Flash, arc or contact.

a. Contact burns
  - Commonest type of injury.
  - This is due to contact with a high voltage system converting electrical energy into heat resulting in tissue damage.
  - The current enters, traverses the body and exits at another site.
  - The final damage depends on the pathway of the current through the body.

b. **Flash burns**—The flash sets the clothing on fire and are usually superficial and heals spontaneously.

c. **Arc burns** give rise to localized deep burns due to intense heat at the termination of current flow.

The current exists and re-enters skin over a fixed joint to find the shortest pathway commonly seen on flexor surfaces of the body.

Pathophysiology of Systemic Changes

- Current passes through the tissues
- Heat is generated because tissue is not a perfect conductor and acts as a resistance.
- The vessels and nerves are good conductors of current while dry skin and bone are poor conductors.
- Immediately after electric shock patient may go into cardiac arrest or develop arrhythmias.
- Due to vascular endothelial damage there may be occlusion, thrombosis and progressive ischemia of the muscles.

Clinical Features

- Depends on mode of injury and duration of contact.
- If patient has been thrown away or has had a fall, internal injury and fracture should be suspected and excluded.
- A crush type of syndrome is seen in the presence of significant amount of dead muscle, this poses a risk of renal failure with the precipitation of muscle break down products like myoglobin and hemoglobin.
- If myoglobinuria persists for more than 6 hours—it is a sign of major muscle loss requiring amputation or debridement.

Management

Emergency first aid is to disconnect from electrical supply by switching off the power as early as possible.

- **Rescue**—Caution must be exercised by the rescuer so that he does not become a part of the electrical circuit in attempting to free a person still in contact with the live wire.
- Use dry wood and push the victim away from current source (Please note if while the power is on and attempt is made to remove the person it can be dangerous to the rescuer as the current can arc as he approaches the victim).
- Take the patient to hospital for further management.
- Cardiac and respiratory status are assessed, ECG should be taken to check arrhythmias.

Resuscitation

- Calculating IV fluid is difficult in electrical burns but the aim should be to clear the pigments like myoglobin and hemoglobin.
- Some advocate 7 ml/kg/% of burns.
- It is important to maintain adequate organ tissue perfusion.
- If adequate fluids are not given, the chances that the patient would go in for renal failure is high. This is due to the pigments which are break down products of dead muscle, leading to damage of the kidneys.
- Some advocate soda bicarbonate infusion in doses of 12.5 gms as IV bolus followed by 12.5 gms per hour to maintain urine in alkaline range to prevent pigment precipitation in renal tubules.

- Urine output should be clear and maintained at 70-100 ml /hour.
- Forced diuresis with mannitol can also be tried.
- Tetanus toxoid is given prophylactically.
- If vascular impairment is noticed due to compartment syndrome fasciotomy should be done immediately.

Surgical intervention - Escharotomy and fasciotomy are frequently required to decompress the tense compartment.

- Initial debridement should be aggressive as non viable tissue left behind can result in infection.
- Early excision and skin grafting should be done if tendons and bones are exposed. Charred extremities should be amputated as early as possible.

Complications

- CNS - loss of consciousness.
- Cardiac - ventricular fibrillation and cardiac arrest.
- Injury to spinal cord with deficits ranging from localized paresis, paralysis to quadriplegia.

Rehabilitation

- The devastating nature of injury makes rehabilitation very important.
- Long term sequelae includes muscle fibrosis and peripheral neuropathy which needs a lot of physiotherapy.

Role of Nurse in Monitoring a Patient with Electrical Burns

- Monitor cardiac status –for irregular heart beats.
- Maintain a clear urine output (to give large amounts of fluid).
- Elevate the burned extremities.
- To watch for sudden arterial blow out leading to massive bleeding and death
  - Immediate compression of the bleeding site with tight bandage
  - Get help and start IV line
  - Inform the doctors
  - Send blood samples for cross match.

Chemical Burns

- A chemical burn is unique because of continuous tissue damaging effect by the chemical till it is completely washed off or neutralized.
- It may be accidental or homicidal.
- The extent of damage is directly proportional to its concentration, volume and the duration of contact.
- Burns generally involve the face and eyes. The color of the skin is dark brown and black. The eschar appears dry, adherent and insensitive to touch.
- It usually involves people at home , industrial workers and those that are involved in chemical warfare.
- The acid trickles down from the face, although the extent of injury is small, the destruction and deformity are severe.

First Aid Management

- Immediately remove all clothes and start continuous copious irrigation with water for at least 30 minutes.
- Early excisional surgery is necessary as spontaneous eschar separation is delayed due to late development of subeschar infection.
- Eye burns should be irrigated with water for a prolonged period of time and an ophthalmologist should be called in as early as possible for expert opinion to prevent blindness.

Frost Bite

Usually involves hands, feet, nose and ears. It is common in unconscious patients.

Classification

Depending on the tissue destruction, it is classified into four degrees:

- **First degree :** Involves superficial skin with edema and hyperemia.
- **Second degree:** Superficial skin injury with pain, paresthesia and vesicle formation.
- **Third degree :** Necrosis of skin.
- **Fourth degree:** Necrosis extends to deeper tissue.

Freezing

It can be either.

- **Rapid:** Where it causes damage and death of the cells due to intracellular injury.
- **Slow:** Freezing which causes extracellular damage leading to dehydration from osmotic fluid shift out of cells.
- **Thawing :** Causes capillary leak and occlusion which leads to edema formation and ischemia.
- **Treatment :** Rewarming, elevation of affected part and prevention of infection.

Chapter 6

INITIAL CARE

First Aid

- Stop the burning process – It depends on the type of burns – like thermal, electrical or chemical.
- The object of first aid is to extinguish the flames and bring down the temperature to normal as early as possible.
- The damage is directly proportional to the temperature of the burning agent and to the duration of contact.
- A person whose clothes are on fire should not run as it fans the flames. The oxygen supply in the air aggrevates the burning process.
- Cover the wound.
- Transport to the hospital.

Treatment at the Scene

Thermal burns: Water is the best option to put off the fire–if water is not available then falling down on the floor and rolling over a blanket may be useful. If nothing is available then roll on the floor or anything that is available to put off the fire. Once the fire is put out remove the clothes to reduce the amount of heat delivered to the body.

The advantage of pouring water

- It is to cool the burn surface and to prevent further destruction of deeper tissues.
- It stabilizes skin mast cells which decrease histamine release thereby decreases edema of the wound.
- It also controls pain.
- Once the fire is put out, remove the burnt clothes, cover the burn wound with a clean sheet and transport the victim to the nearest hospital.

1. **Chemical burns:** Large amounts of water should be used to wash away the chemicals . Washing will not only reduce the deeper destruction of tissues, but will also reduce the chances of toxic effects due to absorption.

2. **Electrical burns:** Switch off the electric supply and remove the victim away from the source of current by using a wooden stick. Monitor the patient for both respiratory and cardiac arrest . Look for associated injuries like fractures, chest injuries and abdominal injuries.

Initial Management

Admission Criteria

Patients who need admission to the burn unit are

- Those with extremes of age.
- Burns more than 15 %.
- Burns involving face, palms, soles and genitalia.
- Chemical burns.
- Electrical burns.
- Inhalation burns.

Reception

- Obtain pertinent history – Time of injury and cause of injury.
- Start intravenous line.
- Calculate fluid needs and adjust infusion rate.
- Insert urinary catheter and monitor hourly urine output of 0.5-1 ml/hour.
- Start nasogastric feeds.
- Determine extent and depth of burns.
- Intravenous analgesics.
- Tetanus toxoid 0.5 ml IM.
- Tetglobe 250 units IM.
- Systemic antibiotics – Intravenous injection of 10 lacs crystalline penicillin every four hours after a test dose.
- Draw blood samples for basic investigations like PCV, BBVS, (blood borne virus studies), serum electrolytes like NA, K and HCO_3, creatinine, and RBS, serum protein, albumin.
- Check the weight/approximate weight.

- Calculate the percentage of burns by Wallace Rule of Nine.
- Monitor- temperature, pulse, respiratory rate, oxygen saturation.

Assessment

Calculate the percentage of burns (Estimating burn size)

- **Children** under 12 years of age **"Lund and Browder's"** formula chart is used to estimate the total body surface area burn involved.
- **Adults-** Wallace's "**Rule of Nines**" is commonly used. According to this head and neck constitute 9% of TBSA, each upper extremity is 9%, each lower extremity is 18 % and anterior and posterior trunk are 18 % each, and 1 % for the genitalia.

  For all age groups **palmar surface** of the patient's hand represents 1% of TBSA burns.

Associated Injury

Evaluate the patient from head to foot for other injuries like spine and abdomen

Treatment: Early coverage of the wounds for second degree burns and early excision of third degree burns with auto skin cover using grafts, and with occasional use of homograft play a crucial role.

- The ultimate goal for all burns is to allow for the wound to heal with the least amount of scarring.
- The management of the burn wound depends on the depth of injury. Each type of burn wound should have a different management strategy.
- **First degree burns** do not require any form of treatment other than possibly a moisturizer.
- **Superficial partial thickness burns** have lost the epidermis but have an adequate density of skin adnexa (hair follicle, sweat and sebaceous glands) to re-epithelialize the wound. A partial thickness burn wound that heals within 2-3 weeks would not be expected to result in significant scarring. Second degree burn that take longer than 2-3 weeks to heal frequently develop hypertrophic scarring. Therefore the goal of treating these superficial wounds is to optimize the extent of re-epithelialization to allow the wound to heal as fast as possible. Skin substitutes play a major role in this group of patients.

- **Deep partial thickness burns** can be treated by early excision and grafting. Upto 20 % can be treated at one time. This way of treatment decreases length of stay and early return to work with less hypertrophic scarring compared with conventional non operative management.

- **Full thickness burns** require different treatment strategies because the wounds will not re-epithelialize unless they are very small. Topical agents used is to minimize bacterial colonization until grafting occurs. Deep burns of any size will scar less if they are treated using early excision and grafting.

- There are two approaches to surgical excision of the burn wound. *Fascial excision*—involves excising the burned tissue including full thickness of investing fascia. The advantages of fascial excision include an easily defined well vascularized plane that readily accepts a graft. The drawback is that healthy viable subcutaneous tissue and dermal elements including lymphatics are included in the excision. Fascial excision causes contour deformities and often lymphedema.

- On the other hand *tangential excision* removes necrotic tissue while preserving as much of the underlying viable tissue as possible. Body contour are better preserved than fascial excision. Diffuse punctate bleeding is the hallmark of a viable wound bed. The points of capillary and arteriolar bleeding are closer together in the upper papillary dermis and more widely separated in the deeper reticular dermis and subcutaneous adipose tissue. The main disadvantage of tangential excision is blood loss, which can be controlled by either application of topical epinephrine or subcutaneous infiltration of vasoconstrictors or use of tourniquets.

- **Topical antibiotics**—The most common broad spectrum topical cream such as *silver sulfadiazine* is used to minimize bacterial colonization. The cream was introduced in 1970s and it continues to be the most popular cream for the treatment of burns. The active component is a mixture of silver nitrate and sodium sulfadiazine. It is very soothing and has broad antimicrobial coverage. Disadvantages of silver sulfadiazine is that it should not be used in patients who have sulfa allergies. It may turn a grey color, but does not stain clothes. It impairs re-epithelialization, so its use for superficial burns is questionable. It leaves a whitish yellowish to greenish exudates on the wound. It also causes brief leukopenia that occurs 3-5 days after the burn.

- **Mupiricin**—It is a popular topical agent for MRSA infection. It can be used intranasally to treat carriers of MRSA.
- **Povidone-iodine solution** –It is an antiseptic used to prepare surgical wounds. It has a broad spectrum of activity covering gram positive, gram negative bacteria , yeast and fungi . It can cause contact dermatitis in some patients.
- **Sodium hypochlorite (dakins solution)**— It is another topical agent with 0.5% or 0.25% sodium hypochlorite which is essentially dilute bleach. Dakins solution has efficacy against bacteria, fungi, and viruses.
- Topical antimicrobial agents have been used for decades to successfully decrease the bacterial load in wounds. Fortunately early excision and grafting of the burn wound has replaced the need for prolonged use of these agents.

General Nursing Care

- Initially sponge bath should be given to maintain hygiene, gradually encourage regular daily baths before dressing.
- Early ambulation is important to prevent wasting of muscles and lung complications.
- Shave scalp hair to prevent infection.
- Apply glycerin to the lips to prevent cracking.
- Clean indwelling urinary catheter frequently and change to a new catheter every week.

Members of The Burn Team

- Burn surgeons
- Burn nurses
- Anesthesiologist
- Respiratory therapist
- Dietician
- Psychologists
- Social workers
- Microbiologists
- Rehabilitation therapists.

Nursing staff form the largest section of the multidisciplinary burn team, responsible for implementing the daily continuous care of the burn patient. Severely burned patients can be very challenging to care for, requiring intensive support physically and emotionally. Burn nurses require a range of skills including management of acutely unwell critical care patients on mechanical ventilation and renal support, sophisticated wound dressing techniques, emotional support for patients and their families.

Nurses on a burn critical care unit will often be the first to spot and bring attention to any changes in the condition of a patient and institute remedial action Because of the nature of injury, burn patients often require a prolonged period of recovery both in the acute and rehabilitative phases . Continuity of nursing staff for patients allows trusting relationship and bonds to develop.

Chapter

7 CLASSIFICATION OF BURNS

Type of Burns

- Flame – Dry heat (when clothes catch fire)
- Scald burns –Hot liquids
- Chemical –Acids and alkali
- Electrical – Flash, contact, arc.

Extent of Burn

1. **Lund and Browder**—the percentage of burns in children is calculated by using this formula.
2. **Wallace's "Rule of Nines"**—is used to calculate the percentage of burns in adults.
3. **Palm of the patient**— is calculated as one percent.

Depth of Burn

The depth of burn determines the type of healing besides being a prognostic factor. Burn wounds are classified according to Boyer into three degrees

- **First degree**
- **Second-** Second degree superficial. Second degree deep.
- **Third degree.**

Chapter

8 PATHOPHYSIOLOGY OF BURN SHOCK

Following burn injury the skin and the deeper structures are destroyed by heat resulting in increased capillary permeability leading to fluid, electrolytes and protein leak from the intravascular to interstitial space.

Inadequate volume resuscitation will produce hypovolemia, resulting in low cardiac output and inadequate tissue perfusion. The goal of resuscitation is to maintain vital organ function, the best guide of adequate resuscitation is the hourly urine output of 0.5 ml/kg/hour.

Stress following burns results in increased oxidation of fat leading to marked weight loss. In addition the loss of appetite leads to poor oral intake resulting in continuous loss of weight. Protein calorie started early prevents this severe catabolic state and has proved to be safe and well tolerated.

The morbidity and mortality have reduced considerably over the past few years. This is due to better understanding and management in terms of initial fluid resuscitation, respiratory care, control of infection with topical and systemic antibiotics, early wound coverage with various biological and synthetic cover and nutritional support with enteral and parenteral hyper alimentation.

a. Burn shock

- Burn shock is both hypovolemic and cellular and is characterized by specific hemodynamic changes
- Decreased cardiac output,
- Decreased plasma volume
- Decreased urine output
- Increased extracellular fluid,

- Increased edema.
- The primary goal is to restore and preserve tissue perfusion in order to avoid ischemia.

Pathophysiology of burn shock is summarized as follows

- Loss of cutaneous barrier function with increase loss of fluid–water loss.
- Altered capillary permeability–protein loss.
- Increased hematocrit–hemoconcentration.
- Destruction of Red cells–blood loss.

b. Changes at vascular level

- After a burn injury there is an increase in the capillary permeability and this is due to the inflammatory mediators.
- Plasma leaks out of the blood vessel into the tissues.
- The leak is maximum in the first 8 hours after burn injury.
- Capillary permeability returns to normal by 36-48 hours.

c. Changes at cellular level

- There is an increase in intracellular sodium concentration and a cellular swelling.
- If resuscitation is inadequate cell membrane potential decreases resulting in cellular death.
- So resuscitation is very important not only to correct hypovolemia but also to prevent cellular death.

d. Changes at tissue level

- Injury to the tissue results in release of metabolic acid substance into the circulation.
- Decreased blood supply results in reduced tissue perfusion leading to poor oxygen.
- If well resuscitated with fluids, the capillary permeability recovers its tone, fluid is reabsorbed and diuresis occurs.
- On the other hand if not resuscitated well, patient goes into shock leading to decreased blood flow to various organs like kidney, heart, skin and intestine.
- Decreased blood flow to skin can result in skin becoming pale. The capillaries passively dilate and fill with blood which becomes deoxygenated and gives blue color to the skin.

- Decreased blood flow to intestine results in passive dilation. Absorption stops leading to vomiting. Decreased microcirculation results in erosion, ulceration and bleeding.

Post burn pathophysiology is divided into 3 periods

I. Resuscitative period –(0-36 hours)

a. **Management:** Airway and pulmonary support particularly if there is smoke inhalation injury.

b. **Cardiovascular support:** Massive fluid losses from a skin burn are the result of 3 processes:
   - Alteration in vascular permeability due to vasoactive mediators.
   - Initial fluid shift due to negative interstitial pressure.
   - Fluid shift into non burn interstitium as a result of burn induced hypoproteinemia.

c. **Wound management:** Assessing the size and depth.

II. Post resuscitative period (2-5 days)

- Ideal time to initiate aggressive wound excision and closure.
- Provide airway and pulmonary support.

III. Inflammation and infection period (6 days to till wound closure)

- The hypermetabolic response to injury begins at about 4-5 days after injury and peaks at about 7-10 days.

Systemic Response to Local Injury

a. Cardiovascular response

- Immediately following burns there is an increase in capillary permeability resulting in decreased cardiac output and decreased blood flow to various organs.
- The loss of fluid continues at a rapid rate for some hours and then gradually decreases in a day or two.
- Capillaries recover their tone and permeability resulting in reabsorption of the edema fluid leading to diuresis.

b. **Renal:** Urine output is reduced due to hypovolemia. Increased amounts of myoglobin and hemoglobin and other toxic products cause decreased output.

c. **Respiratory system**

- In hypovolemic shock phase, respiration becomes shallow and rapid due to lactic acidosis.
- Circumferential burns on the chest may lead to shallow breathing resulting in hypoxia.
- Infection leads to ARDS but the more likely cause is due to inflammatory mediators from the burn wound. This explains early respiratory signs even before infection sets in.
- Burn lung syndrome is insidious in onset. Manifests within 2-5 days and the first symptom is increased respiratory rate, difficulty in breathing, rales and ronchi.

d. **Hematologic changes:** Altered capillary permeability allows loss of protein and electrolyte leading to hemoconcentration. **Anemia** seen after burn injury at the end of first week is due to

- Red cell destruction as a result of injury.
- Damaged red cell agglutination, and inactivation by sludging phenomenon.
- Accelerated rate of hemolysis from increased red cell fragility.
- Reduces half life of red blood cells.
- Reduced nutrition leads to reduced hemopoietic production.
- Thrombosis of blood in capillaries in the burned areas.
- Loss through wound donor site.
- Hemolysis associated with septicemia.
- Wound debridement and daily dressing.

Significant changes occur in the red cell and in the clotting system following burn injury. Initially there are elevated levels of hemoglobin because of massive plasma loss. There is also red cell destruction due to direct heat. The life span of RBC is also shortened due to circulating factors. All this leads to progressive anemia during the end of first week.

e. **Gastrointestinal system**

- Hypovolemia can result in splanchnic vasoconstriction leading to paralytic ileus.
- Bowel movement returns to normal after resuscitation.
- Impairment of normal gut mucosa barrier function may occur allowing gut bacteria and toxins to translocate from the lumen

to the lymphatics and mesenteric lymph nodes finally gaining access into blood producing sepsis.

f. **Musculoskeletal system:** Cell membrane gets damaged by burns and myoglobin is released from muscle cells. Muscle wasting and osteoporosis may occur due to prolonged immobilization.

g. **Immune system:** Injury damages the skin barrier function. Suppression of both the cellular and humoral immunity leads to immunosuppression in burn victims.

Normally skin provides the first barrier to bacterial invasion. Its normal excretion of sebum further provides bactericidal properties. Burning removes outer layer. All proteins are depleted in the first week following burns.

h. **Metabolic nutritional response:** Various hypermetabolic responses like

- Increased oxygen consumption,
- Increased energy expenditure,
- Increased rate of lipolysis,
- Increased protein catabolism
- Increased nitrogen loss are seen.

Increased water loss results in cooling of body and shivering leading to additional heat expenditure. Hence use of air conditioning burn units are to be avoided.

Protein metabolism: Following burns the urinary nitrogen begins to increase in levels of 2-3 times normal urinary excretion and the patient remains in negative nitrogen balance which continues until wounds are closed.

Since the main source of this nitrogen appears to be from skeletal muscle extreme degree of muscle wasting can be seen if vigorous attempts to maintain adequate protein and nitrogen are not accomplished. Low protein is also responsible for delayed healing and poor graft take.

Protein loss can be from

- Loss in initial burn wound
- Reduced protein intake
- Continued loss from burn area
- Increased excretion of urinary nitrogen
- Infection.

Carbohydrate metabolism: Hyperglycemia and glucosuria may occur as the balance of insulin is disturbed. There also appears to be insulin inhibition and resistance.

- Fat and vitamins - Increased oxidation of fat in response to trauma is one factor for weight loss.
- **In summary the pathophysiology of burn injury can have two types of effect:** One local and the other systemic effects

  1. **Local effects:** Inflammatory mediators are released from capillary wall resulting in vasodilatation and increased capillary permeability leading to fluid loss.

  2. **Systemic effect:** Includes hypovolemia, immunosuppression, catabolism, pulmonary edema and loss of the protective function of the gut

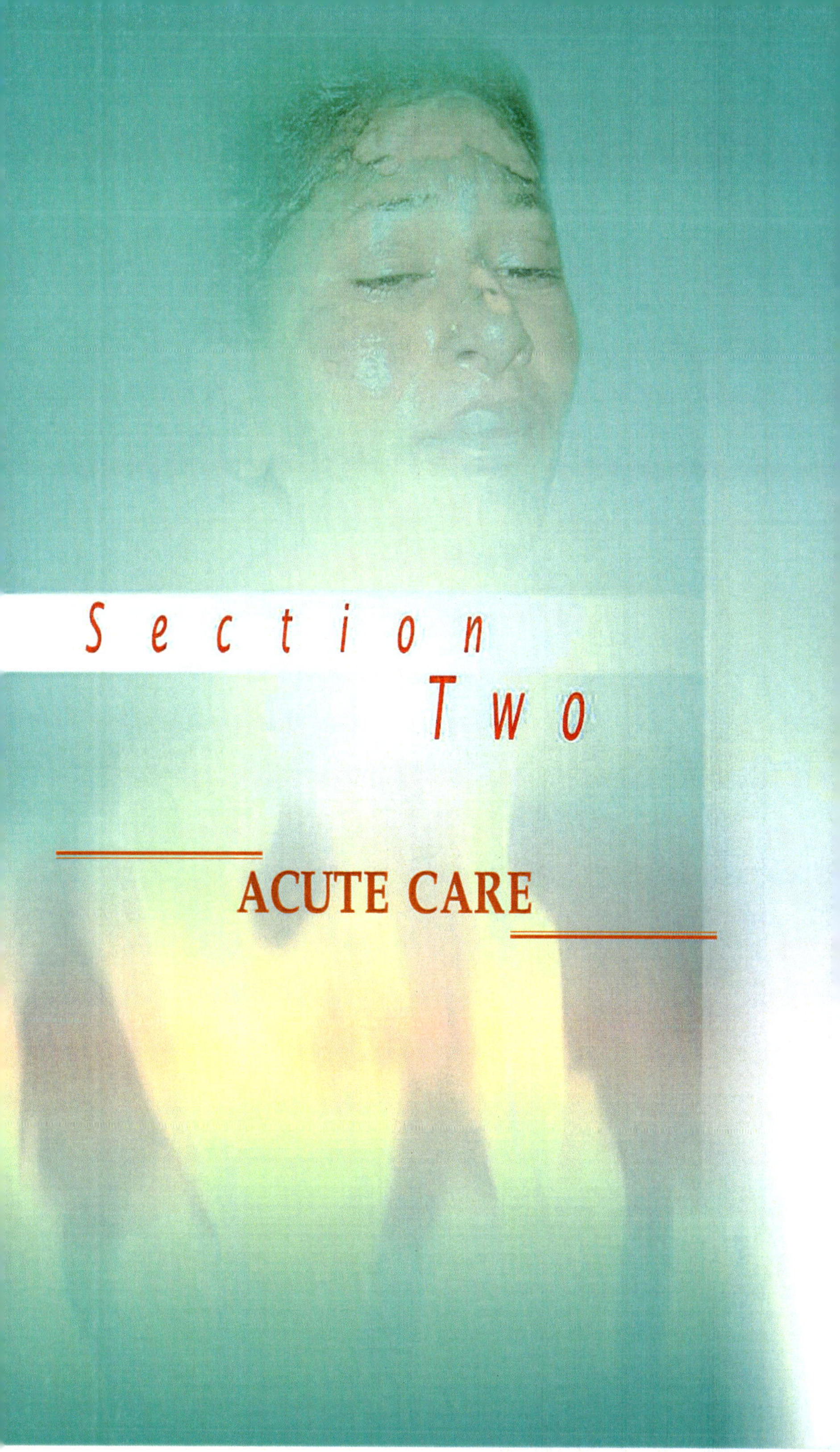

Section Two

ACUTE CARE

Chapter

9 INTRODUCTION

Management at the Scene

- Stop the burning process.
- Put out the fire.
- Remove the victim from the source of injury.
- Remove the clothing and cover with a clean sheet.
- Assess the burn percentage by following "Rule of Nines."

Care of the Burn Wound

- Irrigate with copious amounts of tap water till the pain subsides (about 10-20 minutes).
- Transport the patient in clean dry sheets.
- Do not use ice.
- Do not let the core temperature drop to lower levels.
- Cover the patient with clean and dry sheet.
- Keep the patient warm.
- Inform the receiving hospital.

Referral Criteria

- Burns in very young children and elderly.
- Chemical and electrical injuries.
- Inhalational injuries.
- Burns involving more than 15% of TBSA in adults and 10% in children.

- Burns of the vital areas [face, hand, foot, genitalia].
- Burns requiring fluid resuscitation.
- Associated other trauma, medical conditions.

Assessment of Burn Depth

First Degree

- Erythema or redness
- Dry
- Painful
- Minimal or no edema
- No blisters

Second Degree

- Superficial
    - Red
    - Blistered
    - Very painful
- Deep
    - White
    - Soft and resilient
    - Hair follicles and sweat glands are intact.

Third Degree

- Painless
- Dry and brown
- Leathery eschar
- Thrombosed blood vessals
- Cutaneous hair can be pulled out easily.

Fourth Degree

Clinical features are similar to third degree together with exposed bone, muscle or tendon.

Fluid Resuscitation

Indications

In children with superficial burns of more than 10% or deeper burns of less than 10%.

- In adults with superficial burns of more than 15% or deeper burns of less than 15%.

Resuscitation Formula

- Evan's formula
- Brooke's formula
- Modified brooke's formula
- Parkland formula.

Chapter

10 FLUID RESUSCITATION

In the beginning of twentieth century, fluid resuscitation of extensively burned patients was characteristically too little and or too late and acute renal failure was a frequent occurrence. Early death as a consequences of shock and organ failure was common place in patients with extensive burns.

The Brook Formula (1953)

- A non colloid fluid was emphasized for the first time.
- First 24 hour - 1.5 ml of lactated ringer's solution and only 0.5 ml of colloid containing fluid/Kg body weight/% body surface area burned plus 2000 ml of 5% dextrose.
- The resuscitation fluid prevented the development of burn shock and eliminated acute renal failure in the early post burn period.

Modified Brook Formula

- Recommended infusion of lesser volumes of only crystalloid fluid during the first 24 hours postburn.
- Because of increased capillary permeability colloid containing fluid was retained within the circulation to no greater extent than an equal volume of crystalloid in the first 24 hours postburn.
- When colloids were administered during the first 24 hours there was significantly greater increase in lung water following resuscitation.
- Based on that information the modified Brooke's formula predicts fluid needs for the first 24 hours for adults as 2 ml of LR/Kg body weight/% body surface area burned .
- The success of lesser volume resuscitation which has been associated with a reduced incidence of compartment syndromes

and other manifestations of fluid overload, has prompted revisions of the resuscitation formula from 2-4 ml of LR/Kg/body weight /% body surface area burned to 2 ml.

When the first 48 hours resuscitation period ends, the burn patient is characterized by expansion of total body water as manifested by edema in burned and unburned tissues producing a 15-20% weight gain and expansion of total body sodium mass as a consequence of the infusion of large volumes of salt containing fluid.

- Fluid management is critical to the survival of a burn victim. A number of methods of fluid resuscitation have been advocated.
- The burn shock is not only due to hypovolemia but also influenced by extra cellular sodium depletion.
- It was noted that the edema fluid contains protein in the same proportion as that found in blood, this became the basis for resuscitation with colloid fluid to increase the plasma volume.
- From this, two things become evident, one to give salt solution and the other to give colloid to increase plasma volume.
- Although so many types of fluids are advocated, one thing is clear, that edema fluid is increased by the amount and type of resuscitation fluid. The consensus is to give least amount of fluid necessary to maintain adequate organ perfusion.
- As far as the optimum type of fluid is concerned, replacement of extracellular salt lost into the burned tissue and into the cell is essential for successful resuscitation.
- Colloids should be given at the end of second 24 hour period to maintain the plasma volume.

Types of Fluid

a. Sodium chloride

b. Ringer lactate

c. Colloid

- It is clear that all solutions are effective in restoring tissue perfusion. Initially salt containing solutions should be administered.
- Colloids should be given 24 hrs post injury to increase plasma volume (plasma would leak out before that due to increased capillary permeability).

- The volume of resuscitation fluid infused should be adequate for tissue perfusion and should maintain a urine output of 0.5- 1 ml /kg/hour.
- It is important to emphasize that all of the resuscitaton formulas are only guidelines.
- Resuscitation is completed when there is no further accumulation of edema fluid, which generally occurs between 18-30 hours post burn.
- Maintenance fluid with potassium supplements should be given because of the loss of intracellular potassium during burn shock period.
- The requirements for fluid calculation are weight of patient, percentage of burns and time of burns.

10.1 VARIOUS FORMULAS

1. **Evans** (1952)
   - Day-1: 1ml of colloid and 1ml/kg/% of electrolyte solution+ normal requirement
   - Day-2: 0.5 ml of colloid and 0.5ml/ kg/% of electrolyte solution+ normal requirement
2. **Brooke** (1953)
   - Day-1: 0.5 ml colloid and 1.5 ml/kg/ % of electrolyte solution + normal requirement
   - Day -2: 0.25 ml of colloid and 0.5 ml kg /% of electrolyte solution+ normal requirement
3. **Modified Brooke** (1970)
   - Day-1: colloid nil 2 ml of electrolyte solution + normal requirement
   - Day-2: 0.5 ml of colloid and 1ml of electrolyte solution + normal requirement
4. **Parkland** (1968)
   - Day-1: No colloid, 4 ml of electrolyte solution (No normal requirement)
   - Day-2: 700-2000 ml of colloid and no electrolyte solution (No normal requirement)

10.2 FLUID CALCULATION

Modified Brooke's Formula (Christian Medical College)

First 24 hour: Burn requirement = Weight in kg × percentage of burns × 2 ml

Plus **Normal** requirement = 2500 ml

(normal requirement of 2500 is because of insensible loss like -lungs -500, skin-500 ml, urine-1400 ml, feces-100 ml)

(Example 50 kg × 50 % × 2 = 5000 ml

Normal = 2500 ml

Total = 7500 ml.

Second 24 hour: Burn requirement=Weight in kg × percentage of burns × 1ml

(Half given as colloid and half as crystalloid)

Normal requirement = 2500 ml

Third 24 hour: 5 % D/S 2000 ml plus -N/S 500 ml

Injection KCl 3 gms.

- We calculate the fluid requirement according to modified Brookes formula (weight x percentage of burns x 2) + Normal requirement
- If the percentage of burns is less than 50 % then calculate the fluid requirement accordingly.
- For example if the patient is 50 kg and has 40 % burns then the fluid calculation for the first 24 hours will be

  50 × 40 × 2 (4000 ml) + 2500 ml of normal requirement. So a total of 6500 ml will be given for the first 24 hours which starts from the time of burns and not from the time the patient is seen in the emergency room.
- It is dangerous to expand the interstitial space by more than 50 % of the original size, so 50% should be the limiting factor for calculating the fluid requirement irrespective of size of burns.

  In burns involving more than 50% body surface area the capillary permeability is at its maximum thus affecting both treatment and prognosis and hence calculation should be for 50 % only even if the burns is over 50%.
- Once shock phase subsides, diuresis and mobilization of sodium occurs and urinary output increases.
- The enormous amount of urine output is due to expanded extracellular fluid, which is excreted out once edema subsides.

- Fluid calculation is only a basic guideline.
- The best guideline is hourly urine output of 0.5-1 ml/ kg body weight / hour.
  - If urine output is adequate same amount is continued during the next hour.
  - If urine output is low , fluid is increased by double the amount of deficit
  - If urine output is high reduce the fluid to an amount that is excess of the normal
  - If urine output is high inspite of very low IV intake , do not worry as re-absorption of edema fluid has started
  - If urine output remains low inspite of large amounts of fluid, it indicates that colloid needs to be transfused.
- Catheterize the patient and adjust the IV fluids according to urine output.
- The goals of fluid resuscitation are to restore and maintain adequate tissue perfusion and oxygenation, avoid organ ischemia and to preserve heat injured but viable soft tissue.

10.3 ROLE OF NURSE IN FLUID RESUSCITATION

Although the doctor calculates the fluid requirement according to the formula . It is the duty of the nurse to adjust the rate of infusion to maintain the urine out put at 0.5 ml to 1 ml /kg/ hour (for example if patient weighs 50 kg, then the urine output should be 25 ml- 50 ml every hour).

Please remember that fluid calculation is only a basic guideline and the best guideline to say that the fluid administered is correct is the hourly urine output.

Chapter

11 NUTRITION

11.1 INTRODUCTION

Nutritional support is vital for the successful management of the burn patient and it requires special attention. Early nutritional support has been shown to reduce mortality and hasten the recovery of the patient. Nutritional requirements are higher among burn patients, owing to the hypermetabolic and other pathophysiologic responses that occur after the thermal injury. An aggressive nutritional support is mandatory to provide optimal condition for wound healing, immunocompetence and ultimate well being of the patient. A high protein, high carbohydrate, low fat diet with supplementation of Vitamin A, C, trace elements and zinc are advocated. Nutritional assessment of the patient is necessary for successful implementation and evaluation of the nutritional therapy. The success of nutritional management of the burn patient depends on the committed effort and well co-orinated approach of the burn care team of clinician, dietician, and nurse.

11.2 AIM

- To provide optimum calories and nitrogen through enteral route (Fig. 11.1).
- To maintain premorbid weight
- To evaluate advantages.

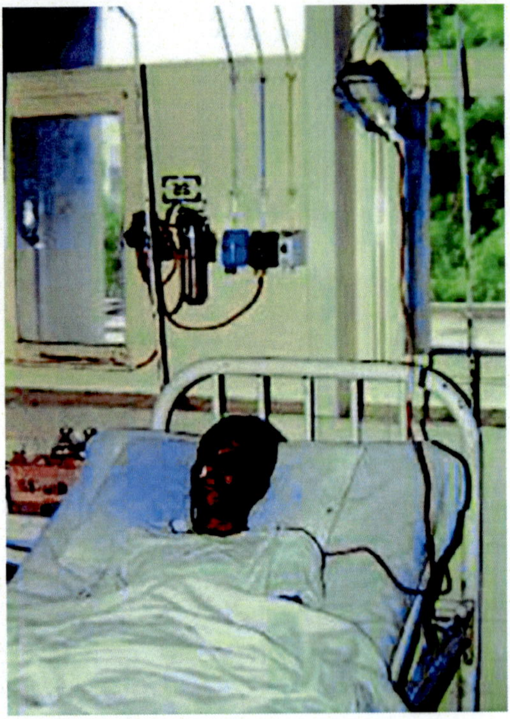

Fig. 11.1: Enteral nutrition supplimentation

11.3 ADVANTAGES

- Wound heals faster.
- Reduces mortality and morbidity.
- Weight gain.
- Short length of hospital stay.
- Less rate of infection.
- Cost effective.
- Improves survival.

11.4 PATHOPHYSIOLOGY

- After burn injury, patients enter into a severe catabolic state characterized by elevated metabolic rate, increased protein mobilization and gluconeogenesis.

- In burn patients these catabolic changes lead to significant increase in energy and protein requirements.
- Weight loss during this phase is virtually inevitable unless aggressive nutritional therapy is instituted soon after the burn.
- Weight loss of more than 10 percent has been shown to increase mortality and a weight loss of more than 30 percent is associated with almost 100 percent mortality). Therefore nutritional support is as important as any other aspect of burn management.
- Nutritional support can be achieved by either enteral or parenteral routes.
- Parenteral nutrition is usually avoided because of its expense and the high rate of complications.
- Nutrition supplementation via a continuous nasogastric tube helps prevent severe weight loss.

11.5 DISTURBANCES IN METABOLISM

- Burns is followed by hypermetabolic response that persists for up to 1-2 years postburn .
- The response is characterized by increased metabolic rates, multiorgan dysfunction, muscle protein degradation, blunted growth, increased risk for infection.
  1. Rise in body temperature.
  2. Endocrine changes consists of elevated catecholamine, corticosteroids and glucagon.
- Management maintain a warm environment, minimize pain, maintain muscle activity, early excision and grafting, early diagnosis of infection and prompt treatment , good nutrition.
- Supplementation of vitamin C to ensure that plasma levels are adequate to support wound healing.
- Blood glucose should be monitored and maintained below 150 mg/dl by use of insulin or dietary adjustments.

Following burn injury there is disturbances of carbohydrate, protein and fat metabolism.

1. **Carbohydrate:** Burn patients have elevated blood glucose levels, this is due to increase glucose production from gluconeogenesis.
2. **Fat:** Increased lipolysis results in increased levels of serum fatty acids.
3. **Protein:** Protein is also altered. Protein break down exceeds synthesis.

There is marked muscle wasting in burn patients.

- Aggressive early enteral feeding improves outcomes in severely burned patients.
- With oral alimentation alone patients loose weight.
- Early enteral nutrition is preferred to parenteral nutrition . Enteral nutrition reduces translocation of bacteremia and sepsis, maintains gut motility and preserves first pass nutrient delivery to the liver.
- Enteral feeding through a feeding tube should be infused continuously and the feeding tube flushed every 8th hourly to prevent inspissations of the feeding mixture.
- Parenteral nutrition should be reserved for those with enteral feeding intolerance or prolonged ileus.
- Daily weights should be obtained to assess the adequacy of diet supplied.

By administering very early nutritional supplementation (VENS) it controls gluconeogenesis, increases glucose utilization and minimizes protein loss. More over it is safe, well tolerated, limits weight loss and controls secretion of catecholamines and glucagon thus reducing hospital stay.

11.6 THE GOALS OF AGGRESSIVE NUTRITIONAL SUPPORT

- Promote early anabolism and wound healing.
- Prevent weight loss.
- Improve immunity.
- To promote wound healing.

- To replace the lost calories and protein.
- To protect body from infection.
- To replace fluid and electrolyte balance.

11.7 EFFECTS OF POOR NUTRITION

- Acute nutritional deficiency.
- Muscle wasting.
- Essential fatty acid deficiency.
- Sever weight loss (Fig. 11.2).
- Liability to increased pressure sore.
- Anemia.
- Poor granulation tissue and delayed wound healing (Fig. 11.3).
- Poor skin graft take.
- Delayed healing of donor site.
- Increased susceptibility to infection.
- Decreased immunological responses.

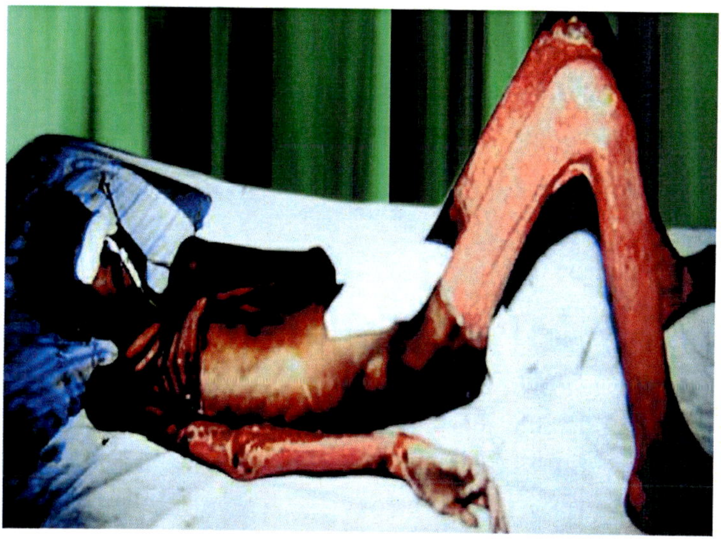

Fig. 11.2: Thin emaciated person with pale wounds

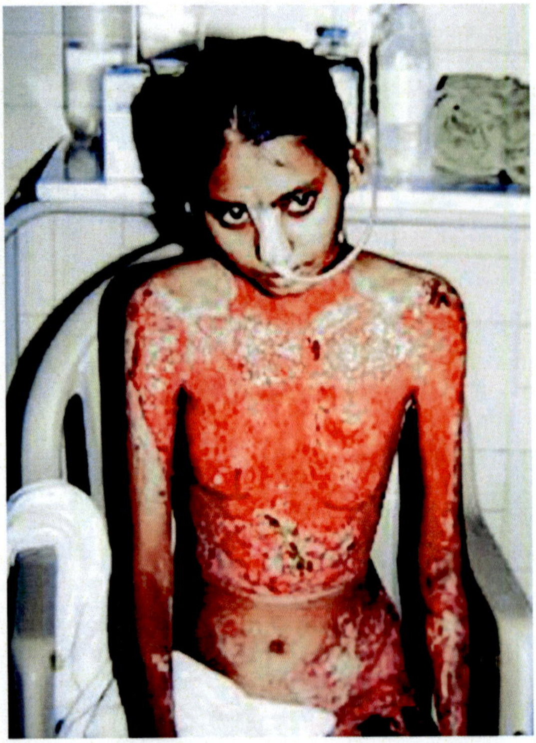

Fig.11.3: Malnutrition with pale wounds

11.8 CHANGES SEEN IN A BURN PATIENT THAT DEMANDS NUTRITIONAL SUPPORT

- Stress response.
- Hypermetabolic response.
- Catabolic response.
- Changes in plasma protein.
- Loss of fat, minerals, trace elements and iron.
- Loss of heat, water and body weight.

11.9 PROBLEMS OF HIGH NUTRITION

Diarrhea: To over come this, enteral nutrition is administered in the form of drip through a nasogastric tube over 24 hours (Fig. 11.4).

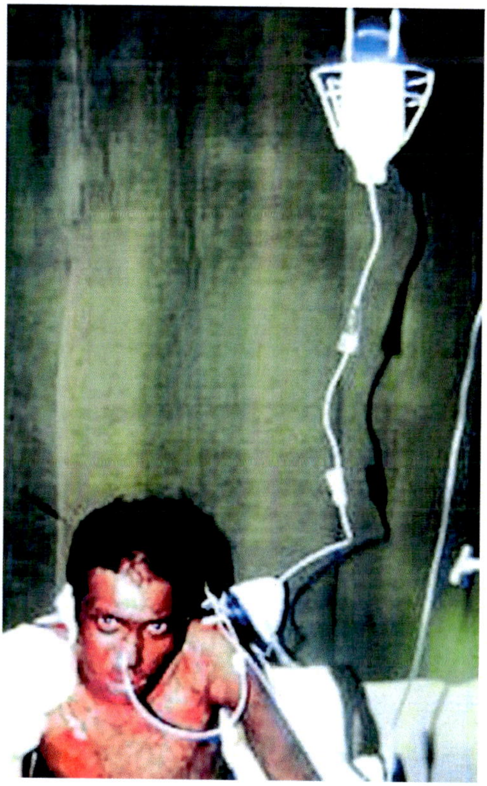

Fig. 11.4: Nutrition in the form of a drip

The clinical outcome and prognosis are influenced by patient's nutritional status.

Importance of early nutritional supplementation to prevent the severe catabolic state is realized.

Simple nutrients like buttermilk should be administered on the first day and gradually increase the strength of the diet. This will help to minimize osmotic diarrhea.

Main problem of feeding via nasogastric tube is diarrhea and vomiting . These should be temporarily managed by decreasing the amount and concentration of feeds or spreading daily feeds over a longer period. If these measures fail give codeine phosphate.

11.10 NUTRITIONAL REQUIREMENT CALCULATION

Determine the calorie and protein needs of a patient by using

Curreri formula = Energy requirement - (25 cal × weight in kg) + (40 cal × % of burns)

Protein- requirement - 3 grams per kilogram

Vitamins and minerals - vit - C -500 mg/day

Vit -K 10 mg/week

Zinc 2-5 mg/day

Trace element solution -10 mg twice a week

- Normal nutrition is necessary to maintain intestinal structure and function.
- To preserve the intestinal mucosal barrier and thereby prevent the translocation of bacteria and endotoxin from the gut to the systemic circulation.
- Nutritional support should be given by enteral route to meet the extra calorie and protein requirement.
- This is achieved by placing a nasogastric tube and giving continuous drip for 24 hours .
- Initially a half strength feed is given gradually building up the full strength feeds over the next few days.

Parenteral is required only when the patient goes into severe sepsis

- Vitamins and minerals are necessary for wound healing and skin maturation.
- Fat-soluble vitamins (A,D,E and K).
- Vitamin C-1000 gms/day should be given for collagen synthesis.
- Vitamin B is needed to metabolize carbohydrate, fat and protein.
- Zinc is essential for DNA synthesis (20% zinc is in the skin).

11.11 ASSESSMENT OF NUTRITIONAL STATUS

- Regular intake and output chart.
- *Physical:* Weight regularly.
- *Immunological:* Total lymphocyte count.
- *Biochemical:* Albumin, serum transferrin level and creatinine.

Evidence of Malnutrition is Calculated by

$$\frac{\text{Usual Wt} - \text{Actual Wt}}{\text{Usual Wt}} \times 100$$

Example if $\frac{60 - 50}{60} \times 100 = 16\%$

(Weight loss more than 10% loss over any given time period has been taken as evidence of malnutrition).

11.12 ROUTES OF NUTRITIONAL SUPPORT

- Oral
- Enteral
- Parenteral

11.13 IMPORTANCE OF VERY EARLY NUTRITION SUPPLEMENTATION

- It not only prevents the severe catabolic state but also influence the clinical outcome and prognosis.
- Simple nutrients like butter milk is given for all burn patients on the first day through a small nasogastric tube.
- From the second day onwards half strength burn formula feeds, gradually increasing the strength to full strength by day three.
- From the 4th day onwards nutrition is calculated according to Curreri formula.
- Parenteral nutrition support like hyperosmolar glucose, amino acids and lipids are given via peripheral line to supplement enteral feeds particularly during sepsis.

11.14 NURSES ROLE IN NUTRITIONAL MANAGEMENT

- Assess age, weight and height.
- Extent and depth of burns.
- Protein and calorie requirement.
- Prepare special feeds and feeding schedule.
- Set specific objectives to attain nutritional status.
- Explain importance of nutrition.
- Minimize stress factors.

- Provide emotional support.
- Maintain good oral hygiene.
- Ensure comfortable position while feeding.

11.15 PLANNING THE DIET

- Calculate the protein and calorie requirement using Curreri formula.
- Normal feeds are given orally and supplements via nasogastric tube.
- Program feeding schedule.
- Observe for food tolerance/symptoms of gastrointestinal tolerance.
- Maintain record of intake/output.
- Maintain weight.
- Encourage early ambulation and activity.
- If patient is on tube feeding proper management of tube feeding is maintained.

11.16 EARLY AND LATE NUTRITIONAL MANAGEMENTS IN CMC

- **Day-I** : Butter milk 50 ml
Q4H aspiration.
- **Day -II** : 1/2 strength burns formula diet.
- **Day-III** : Full strength burn formula diet.
- **Day-IV** : Full strength burn formula with high protein diet.

11.17 COMPOSITION OF BURNS FORMULA DIET (BFD) USED IN CMCH,VELLORE

Ragi Feed

1. Milk : 400 ml
2. Ragi : 80 gm
3. Milk powder : 120 gm
4. Sugar : 40 gm

Total : 1200 ml

Total calories	: 460 cal
Total protein	: 53 gm
Cost	: 38 Rs.

Rice Feed

1. Protinex	: 30 gm
2. Complan	: 120 gm
3. Rice Flour	: 75 gm
4. Milk	: 900 ml
5. Sugar	: 60 gm
Total	: 1200 ml
Calories	: 1750 cal
Protein	: 70 gm
Cost	: 70 Rupees

11.18 ADVANTAGES OF SPECIAL FOOD (BFD)

- Easily digestible
- High protein calorie diet
- Inexpensive
- Easily available
- Fastens healing.

11.19 FACTORS RESPONSIBLE FOR SUCCESS IN NUTRITIONAL MANAGEMENT

- Patients involvement in accepting feeds.
- Prompt assessment and implementation of administrating feeds.
- Frequent evaluation of responses related to feeds.
- Assessing weight, wound healing, bowel pattern and improved investigation values.
- Reporting and documenting.
- Health education of patient and family.

11.20 CONCLUSION

- The high protein calorie diet given very early seems to off set the ravages of hyper metabolism.

- Graft take is good.
- Infection is reduced.
- Patient gains weight (Fig. 11.5)
- Rapid wound healing.

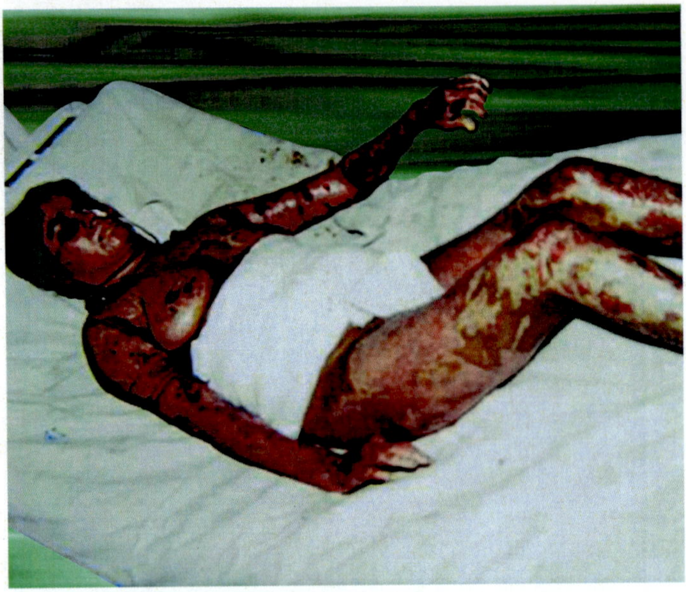

Fig. 11.5: Weight gain due to early nutrition supplimentation

11.21 IMPORTANT POINTS TO NOTE

- Keep the room temperature warm.
- Use occlusive dressing to decrease evaporative water loss.
- Stress affects metabolic rate resulting in muscle and fat wasting and hence dressing change should be quick so as to avoid cold stress.

Chapter

12 BURN WOUND CARE

Burn wound differs from other wounds in the following:

- Area is extensive.
- It is open for long periods and prone for infection.
- It has large amount of dead tissue and discharge from wounds.
- The depth of burn wound depends on the temperature and the duration of contact of the burning agent.

12.1 JACKSONS ZONE OF INJURY

Jacksons zone of injury corresponds to a partial thickness burn (Fig. 12.1).

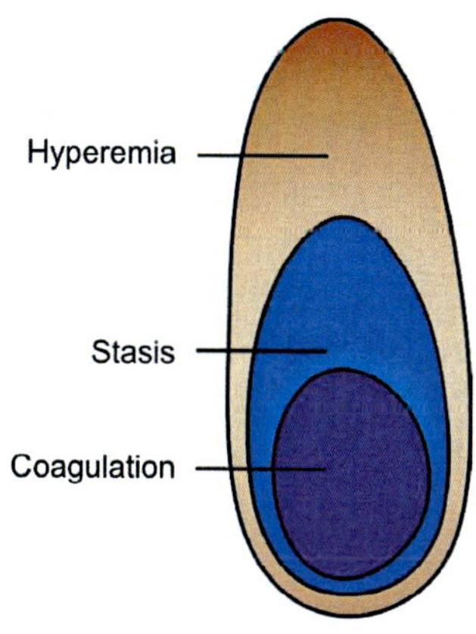

Fig. 12.1: Jackson's zones of injury

Zone of Hyperemia

Minimal injury. This area recovers in 7 to 10 days.

Zone of Stasis

Most cells are initially viable. Circulation becomes progressively impaired leading to cessation of blood flow. This can be reversed if properly resuscitated.

Zone of Coagulation

Central area of burn wound closest to the heat source with coagulation of cells. No blood flow, cells are non viable

- Burn wound is sterile to start with, later it gets infected.
- Bacteria multiplies in the dead tissue producing foul smell.
- Bacteria also invades living cells.
- Toxins are absorbed in the body causing septicemia.
- Systemic and local antibiotics may not reach burn wound as it cannot penetrate dead tissue. So by removing all non viable dead tissue, prevention of wound dehydration and accumulation of purulent secretion an environment conducive to wound healing is achieved.
- Good nutritional support must be provided for early wound healing.

The main aim of local treatment is to minimize toxemia and promote wound healing. As wound gets infected they manifest signs and symptoms of toxemia such as rapid pulse, respiration, high temperature and oliguria. Toxins are released from two sources:

- From bacteria grown on the burned area.
- From products of tissue breakdown.

Burn wounds are either closed spontaneously or closed surgically. Wounds which do not heal in 3 weeks should be skin grafted to avoid scarring, breakdowns and pigmentation.

12.2 TREATMENT OF SUPERFICIAL BURNS

- De-roofing the blister, removing the fluid and retaining the skin is important as the blister fluid contains inflammatory mediators known to be detrimental to the microcirculation in the zone of stasis (Fig. 12.2).

- If blister is already debrided wound should be cleaned and a non-adherent dressing or synthetic dressing applied.
- Wound heals spontaneously in 2 to 3 weeks (Fig. 12.3).
- Wound healing can also be hastened by using biological skin substitutes like biobrane (Figs 12.4 and 12.5).
- Wound healed with Healicoll (Figs 12.6 and 12.7).
- Wounds healed with amnion (Fig. 12.8).
- Superficial burn is suscepitable to sun burn for 1 to 2 years. Patient should be cautioned against pigmentary changes and advised sun protection both physical and chemical. Use of caps, sun protecting factor creams to avoid sun exposure.
- Second degree deep burns
- Second degree deep can heal spontaneously in three weeks (Figs 12.9 and 12.10).
- Second degree deep can also be treated with amnion (Fig. 12.11).
- Second degree deep can also be treated by tangential excision and skin grafting (Fig. 12.12).
- Second degree deep burns can also undergo debridement and skin grafting (Figs 12.13 and 12.14).

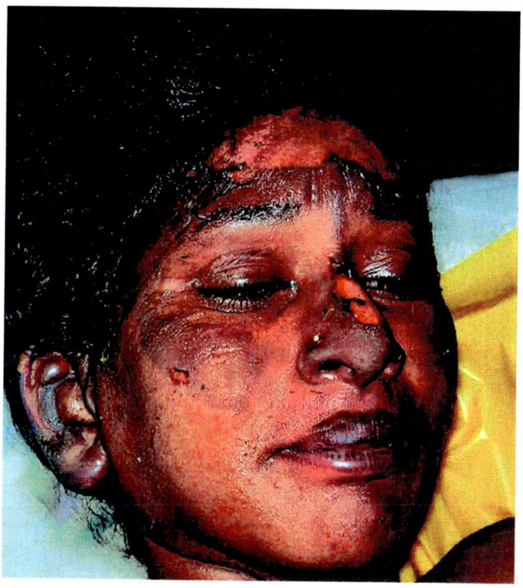

Fig. 12.2: Superficial burns

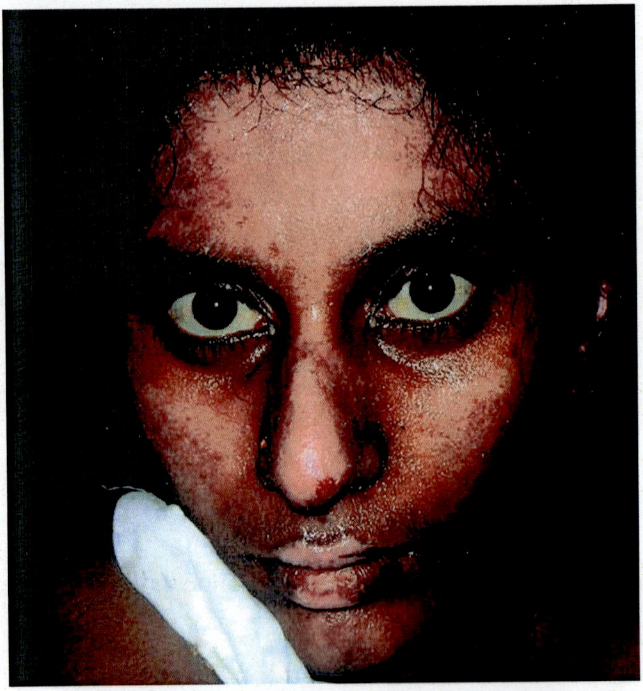

Fig. 12.3: Superficial burns healed spontaneously

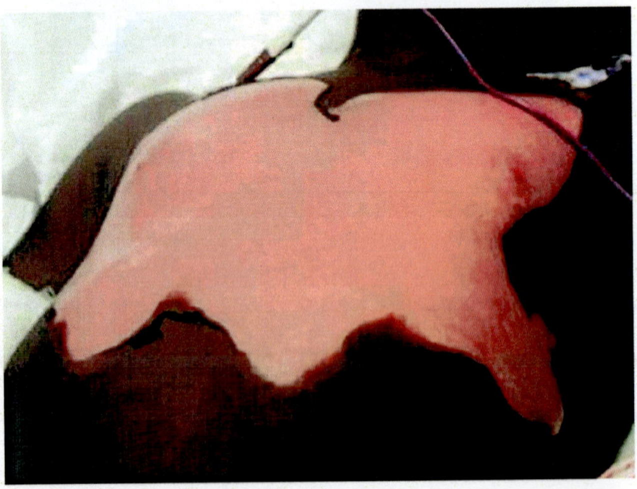

Fig. 12.4: Second degree superficial burns after cleaning

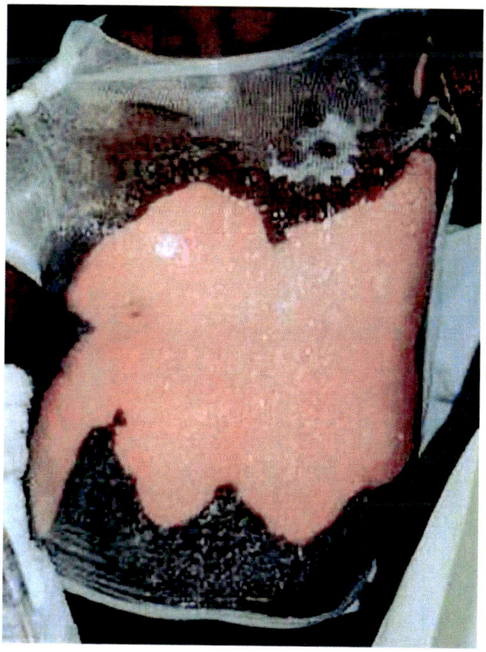

Fig. 12.5: Skin substitute—Biobrane cover for healing

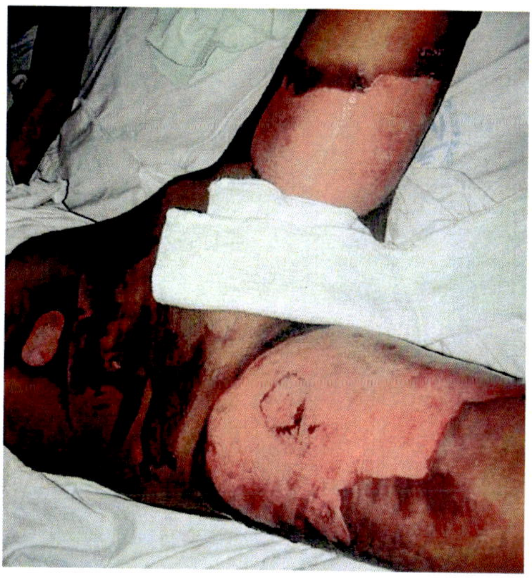

Fig. 12.6: Superficial burns after cleaning

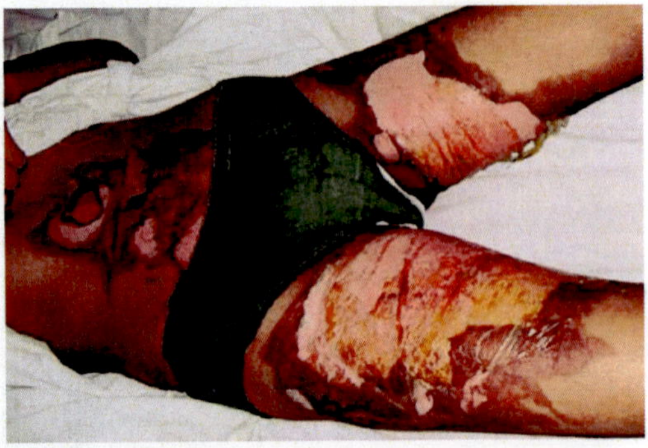

Fig. 12.7: Superficial burns healed with healicoll skin substitute

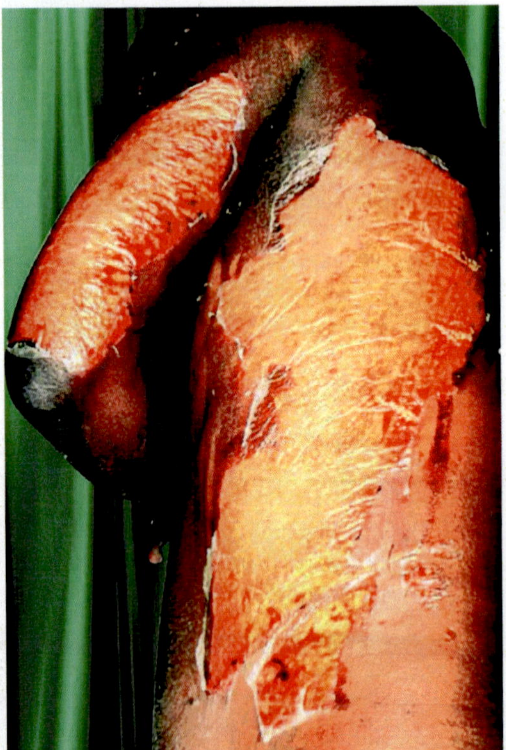

Fig. 12.8: Second degree superficial burn healed with amnion cover

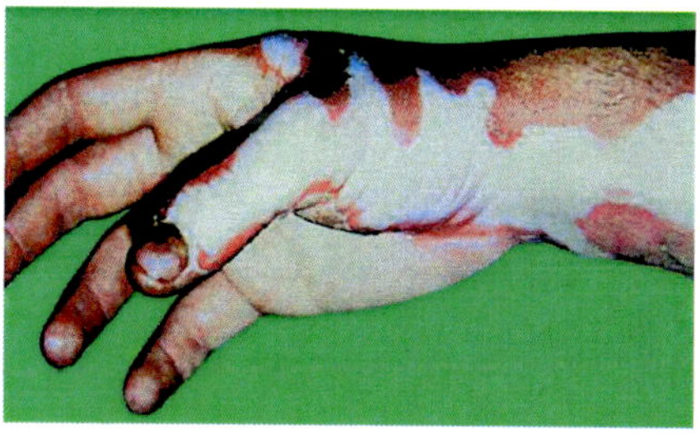

Fig. 12.9: Second degree deep burns showing pink and white appearance

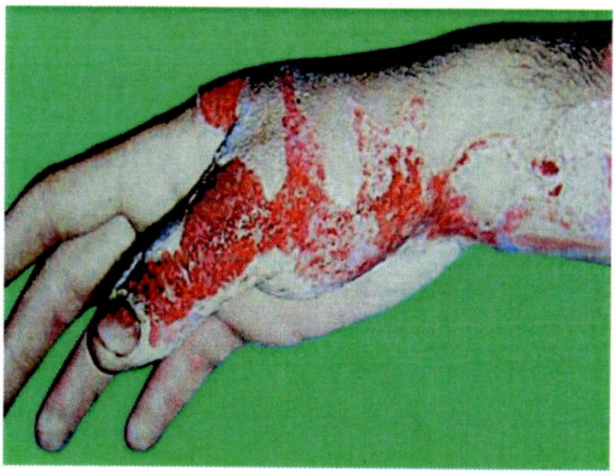

Fig. 12.10: Second degree deep burns healing spontaneously

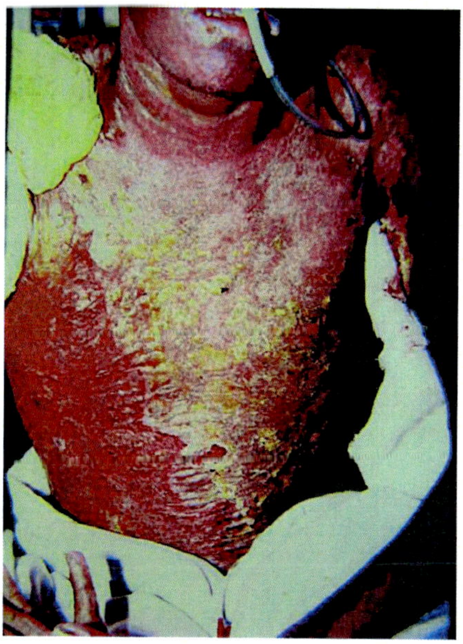

Fig. 12.11: Second degree deep burns healed with amnion

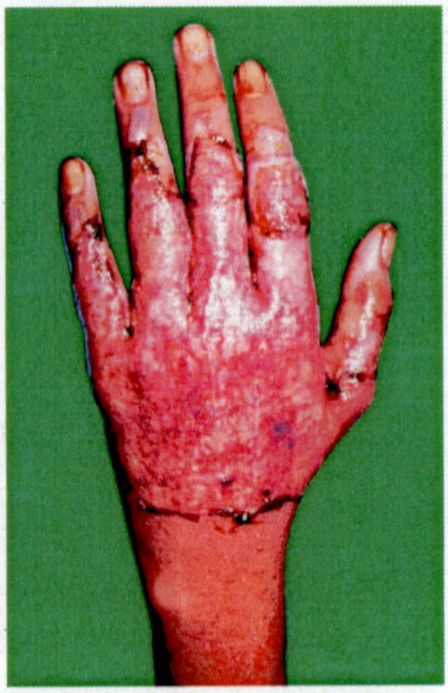

Fig. 12.12: Tangential excison and grafting for second degree burn

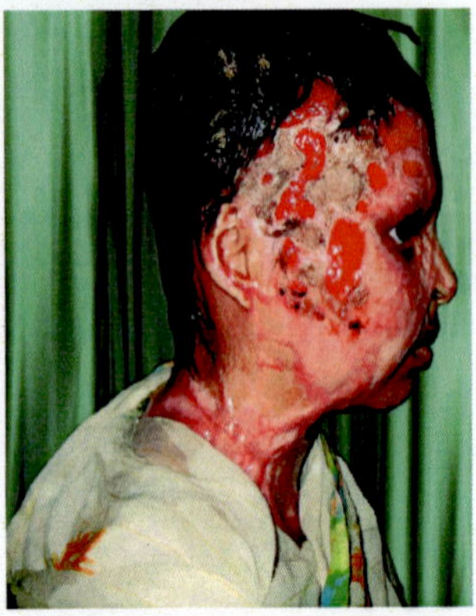

Fig. 12.13: Second degree deep burns showing thin flimsy skin

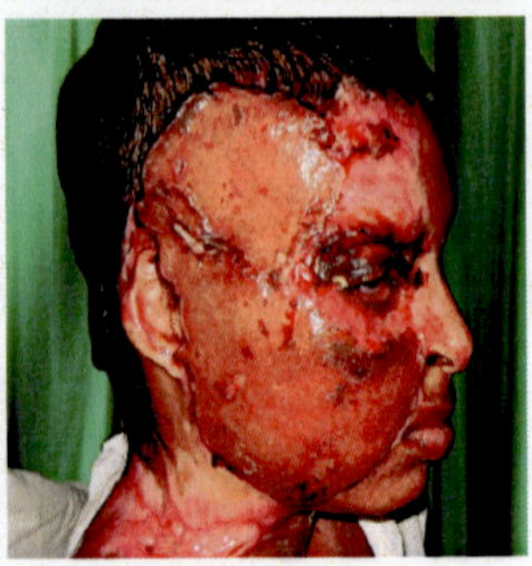

Fig. 12.14: Split thickness skin graft

Consideration in Would Healing

- Hyperpigmentation is a common complication of superficial burn.
- Initially the wound undergoes vasodilatation and hyperpigmentation changes . It is at this stage that care should be given to prevent scarring . The scarring and sequelae are minimized by 6-8 months.
- A deeper second degree burns has a higher chance of hypertrophic scar formation.
- Pressure garments, moisturizing lotions and sun protecting creams are important

12.3 TREATMENT OF FULL THICKNESS BURNS (FIGS 12.15 A TO C)

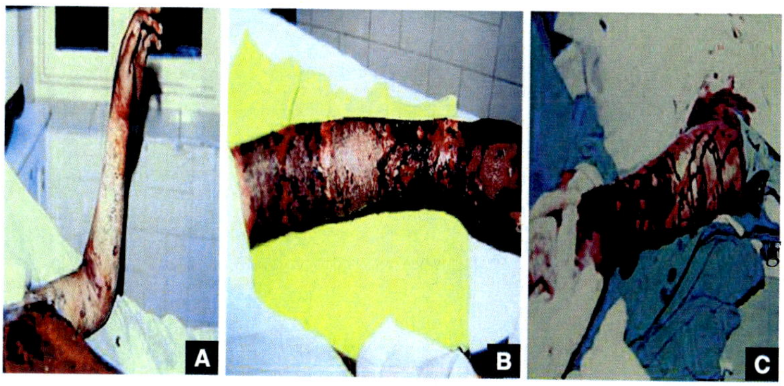

Figs 12.15 A to C: Third degree burns treated with tangential excision and skin grafting

- Complete destruction of all epidermis and dermis.
- Break down of hemoglobin results in many colors on the wound.
- Appearance of skin may be waxy, dry, leathery, charred or translucent. Visible thrombosed veins are seen.
- Prompt burn wound excision and autograft is the best option.

Calculation of Expected Blood Loss at Surgery

If surgery is performed in less than 24 hours from injury -

< 24 hours - 0.45 ml/sq cm burn area.

< 3 days - 0.75 ml/ sq cm burn area.

> 4 days - 0.90 ml/sq cm burn area.

If the burn wound is infected - 1-1.25 ml/sq cm burn area.

Blood Transfusion

Amount of blood should be 1 % of the patients estimated total blood volume for every 1% of full thickness burns

Total blood volume can be estimated by the formula = 80 ml/kg

For example a 50 kg patient has a blood volume of

$$(80 \times 50 = 4000 \text{ ml})$$

If the same patient has FTB of 20% they should receive 20 % of their blood volume which is 800 ml

$$\frac{4000 \times 20}{100} = 800 \text{ ml}$$

12.4 OBJECTIVES OF MANAGEMENT OF BURN WOUND

- Prevent infection.
- Cleaning and removing the dead tissue.
- Preparing the wound for grafting and healing.
- Providing the patient comfort.
- Reducing scarring and contracture.

12.5 TYPES OF DRESSING

Dressing Procedure

- Wear gown , mask and cap.
- Wash hand with soap and water.
- Wear gloves to remove the soiled dressing material, discard the gloves and wear a sterile glove to do the dressing.
- The type , frequency and the amount of dressing depends on the sogginess and infection present.
- As wound starts healing frequency of dressing is reduced.

12.6 TECHNIQUE OF DRESSING

Open Technique

Advantage

- Wound is left open to dry and form an eschar of the necrotic tissue.
- Easy method of management.
- Requires less skill, less people, less time and less cost.

Disadvantage

- Dry tissue.
- Desiccation of the growing epidermis.
- Exposure attracts infection from personnel, visitors insects and flies.
- Infection collects underneath the eschar and septicemia follows.

Closed Technique

Advantage

- Wound covered with adequate dressing using antibiotic ointment and absorbent dressing.
- Biological or synthetic dressing.
- Protects the burn wound from drying , infection and discomfort.

12.7 IMPORTANCE OF DRESSING

- To absorb the burn fluid.
- To protect the wound from the environment.
- To decrease pain.

12.8 DIFFERENT TYPE OF OINTMENT AND DRESSING MATERIAL

1. Silver sulpha diazene (SSD).
2. Betadine.
3. Saline.
4. Jelonet.
5. Banana leaf

Biological Dressing

The aim is to prevent infection, oozing and loss of protein

- Amnion membrane
- Collagen sheet
- Opsite
- Autograft
- Homograft
- Xenograft
- Isograft.

Amniotic Membrane

The amniotic membrane is obtained from fresh placenta. It is separated from the chorion layer of the placenta. It is used to cover the burn wound. Advantage is low cost. Once amnion is applied on the burn wound it is left open and does not require dressing. Amnion is an excellent biological dressing.

Physiological Effects of Amnion

Human amnion has fibronectin —a collagen lattice as well as an epithelial cell layer which can act as a barrier similar to the epidermis. It adheres to the burn wound very well.

Indications

Second degree superficial and deep burn wounds.

Contraindications

- Infected wounds.
- Third degree burns.

Procedure

Amniotic membrane is obtained from a postnatal mother who is free from bio-hazards (seronegative for hepatitis B & C, HIV and syphilis). Amnion is separated from placenta and is washed with saline and stored in glycerol solution. The processed membrane is stored at 4° C in the refrigerator before use.

Advantages

- It is a readily available biological dressing material.
- Not only prevents oozing of plasma from burn wound but also relives pain and controls sepsis.
- Patient requires fewer days of hospitalization.
- Inexpensive and easily available.
- The membrane prevents heat and water loss from the burn wound surface and acts as barrier against bacterial contamination, thus aiding the healing process and reducing the morbidity.
- Practical aspects of this method of treatment can be adopted by any hospital.

Complication

- It has no adverse reaction, and there is a chance for infection if strict aseptic technique is not followed.
- Risk for disease transfer.

Conclusion

- Amnion is easy to handle and sticks well to the raw burn wound bed.
- Once the amnion applied over the burn wound dries , further dressing is not required.
- It reduces pain, heat loss , water loss and gives superior wound healing.

Homograft

Skin used from same species, .i.e. human to human.

Heterograft

From other species, for example from pig.

Synthetic Skin

Artifically produced skin.

Topical Antibiotics

Silversulphadiazine (commonly used).

Advantages

- Bacteriostatic.
- Easy to apply.
- Low toxicity.
- Less painful.
- Infiltrates dead tissue well.

Disadvantages

- Adverse effect on donor site.
- Black staining.
- Transient leukopenia.
- Dilutional hyponatremia.

- Delayed eschar separation.
- Depressed renal function.
- Epithelialization is retarded.

1. **Betadine:** It is bacteriocidal, easy to apply, painful and can cause iodine toxicity.
2. **Neosporine ointment:** It is a combination of bacitracin, polymyxin. It is bacteriocidal and costly.
3. **Circumferential burns:** The leathery eschar produce chest constrictions and compartment syndromes in the extremities or distal ischemia and necrosis.

   Immediate escharotomy/Fasciotomy should be performed in the mid lateral lines of the affected extremities.

12.9 PRINCIPLES OF DRESSING TECHNIQUE

- The main aim of local treatment is to minimize toxemia and promote wound healing.
- Burn wound is cleaned adequately at each dressing and topical antimicrobial agent like 1% silver sulfa diazine cream is applied generously.
- Topical antimicrobial agent is changed in the second week of burns or when burn wound infection is suspected.
- Early excision of dead tissue reduces the chance of bacterial colonization.
- Cover the wound with a dressing that retain the moisture.
- A moist dressing is very comfortable to the patient, prevents desiccation of growing epithelium, relieves pain and permits active and passive movement.
- When ever possible extremities should be elevated to reduce edema.
- Splinting of the extremities may be required.
- Observation should be made at the time of dressing for any change in the wound and immediately brought to the notice of the treating doctor.
- Changes can be foul smelling, color, slough, hemorrhagic spots and blueness of limb.

12.10 TYPE OF BURN WOUND EXCISION

- Early excision of full thickness burn tissue results in better functional and cosmetic effect .
- Tangential excision and autografting with split thickness skin graft.
- Fascial excision performed in very deep full thickness burns results in severe contour deformities.

12.11 ROLE OF NURSE IN BURN WOUND MANAGEMENT

The most important role of a nurse is to indentify the degree of burns, because superficial second degree burns heals spontaneously in 7 days and hence a non adherent gauze impregnated with antibiotic or petroleum dressing should be applied and care should be taken to preserve the growing epithelium.

Deep partial thickness burns starts healing in the second week, care should be taken to avoid infection and injuring the new epithelium.

Third degree burns needs debridement and daily twice dressing to make the wound ready for grafting. Culture sensitivity should be done regularly.

Hemoglobin should be maintained above 10 gms % to minimize invading infection.

12.12 CONCLUSION

Although there are many different types of burn wound, the extent of tissue destruction is always dependent on the temperature, duration of contact and the thickness of the involved skin.

Burns, which are unlikely to heal in less than 3 weeks, should be treated by early excision and grafting.

Postoperative Wound Care

- Graft care with moisturizing cream.
- Splints to prevent flexion contractures.
- Pressure garments to prevent hypertrophic scars.
- Regular exercise both by physiotherapist and occupational therapist.
- Psychological counseling.

Chapter

13 PREPARING THE PATIENT FOR SURGERY

13.1 PREPARING THE PATIENT

- The treatment team will start to prepare the patient for surgery.
- The patient and the family are informed of the plans:
  - The date and time of surgery.
  - Type of surgical procedure.
  - The operation site.
  - Where the skin is taken for grafts.
  - Where the patient can expect most pain in the post operative phase.
- The type of bed, position and whether the patient will need splints postoperatively will be planned before the patient leaves to the operating room.
- The previous evening of surgery—anesthetist will discuss with the patient the type of anesthesia.
- The nurse will make a note of the instruction and advice the patient and the relative about starvation from midnight.

Preparation of the Wound

- The wound is cleaned and a moist dressing (saline dressing) is applied before sending the patient to the operation room.
- Preparation of the donor site:
  - Shave the donor area the previous day.
  - Wash the area with soap and water and apply a sterile towel.

On the Day of Surgery

- Give bath to the patient.
- Make the patient to void.
- Give premedication.
- Pray with the patient and send them to the OR.

Chart Work

- Enter all the details.
- Send IP and OP chart.
- Prescription slip (to enable the doctor to write post op medication).
- Medication - antibiotics to be given per operatively.
- Splints.

After Receiving the Patient from OR

- Check for level of consciousness.
- Check the vital signs like pulse, respiration , BP.
- Check for bleeding.
- Position the patient according to the doctors instruction.
- Check the IV line.
- Strap the urinary catheter.
- Give pain medication.
- Once the patient is made comfortable , go through the chart to see if any specific instructions have been written by the doctor and follow the instruction.

Chapter

14 EMERGENCY SURGICAL PROCEDURES IN BURNS

14.1 DIFFERENT TYPES OF SURGICAL INTERVENTION

- Escharotomy.
- Fasciotomy.
- Excisional surgery - Tangential excision.
- Wound debridement.
- Amputation.

Escharotomy

Deep burns on the chest and extremities lead to constriction. Escharotomies are performed in the ward with sedation. The thick eschar is cut in the form of a grid to relieve this constriction. (Fig. 14.1).

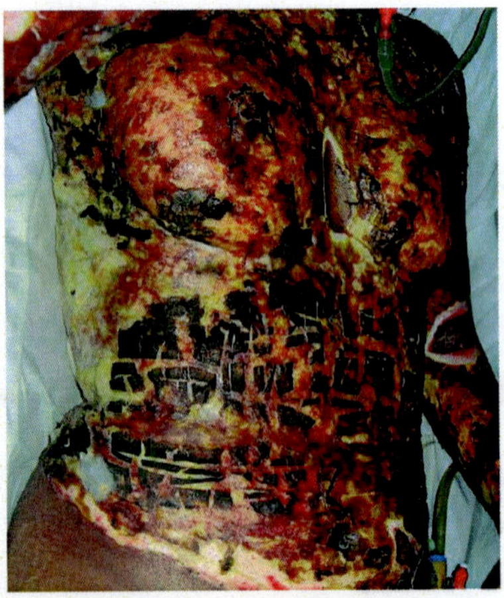

Fig.14.1: Grid escharotomy

Fasciotomy

This is very commonly performed in high voltage electrical burns of the extremities leading to edema and increased compartment syndrome. Fasciotomy is performed in the ward under sedation. The incision is made up to the fascia so that the muscles bulge out of the tight compartment (Fig. 14.2).

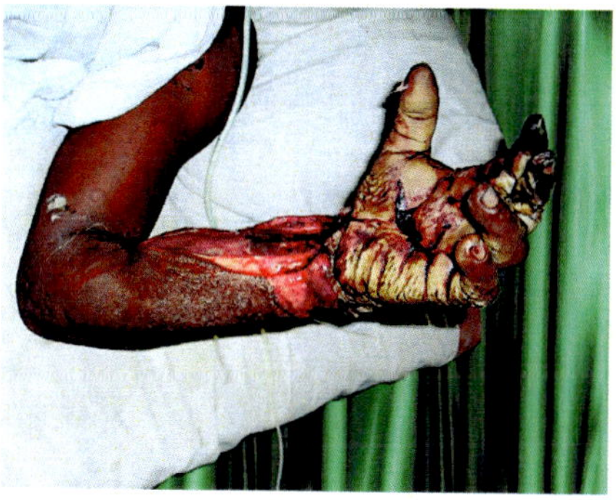

Fig. 14.2: Electrical injury requiring fasciotomy of forearm

Tangential Excision

This is performed in cases where the depth of the burn is question able. It is layer after layer excision of the burn surface till bleeding tissue/viable tissue is seen. Immediate graft has to be laid over the excised area to prevent drying of the wound (Fig. 14.3).

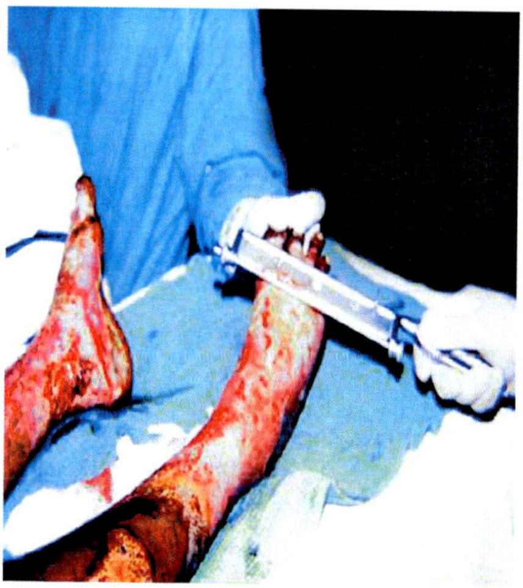

Fig. 14.3: Second degree deep—tangential excision

Wound Debridement

This is done both in the ward and in the operation room to clean the wound for subsequent cover. Either a Humby's knife or 15 blade can be used to debride the slough. Wet dressings help in early removal of slough.

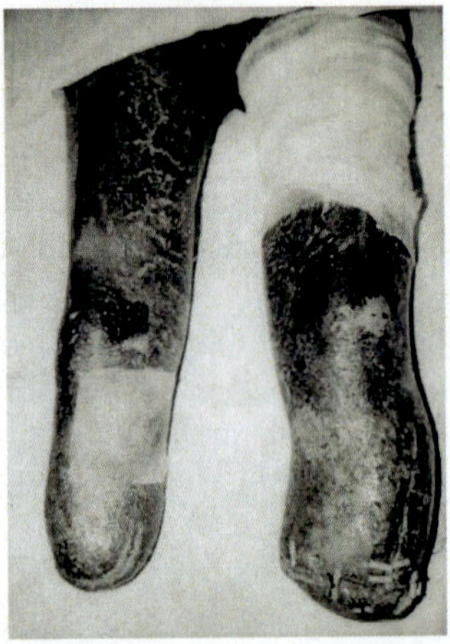

Fig. 14.4: Bilateral below knee amputation

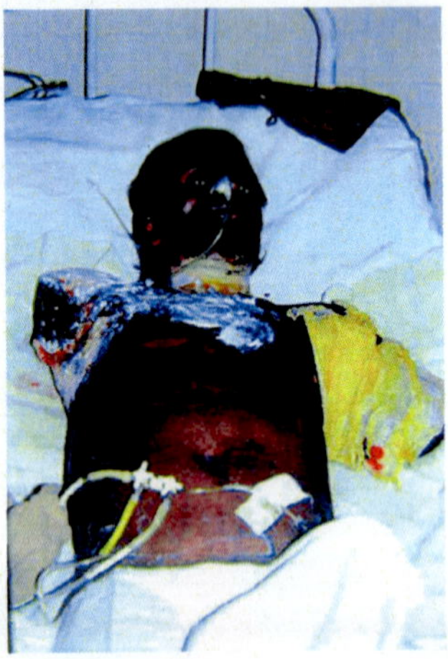

Fig. 14.5: Bilateral amputation

Amputation

In deep burn wounds, inspite of fasiotomy, if gangrene is seen then amputation at various level should be performed (Figs 14.4 and 14.5).

Chapter

15 SKIN GRAFT

15.1 DEFINITION

Graft

Graft is a piece of skin which is completely detached from the body devoid of its blood supply and transplanted to other raw area where it develops a new blood supply for its survival (Figs 15.1 A and B).

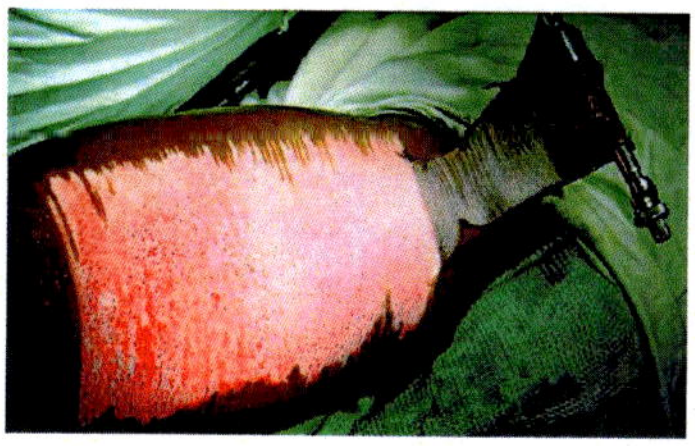

Fig.15.1 A: Skin graft

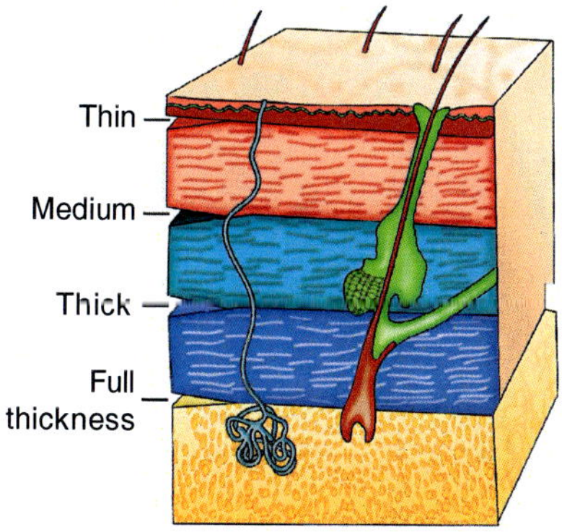

Fig.15.1 B: Level of skin grafts

Donor Area

The area from where the skin graft is removed or harvested is called donor area.

Recipient Area

The area where the graft is applied or laid is called recipient area.

15.2 CLASSIFICATION

Skin graft consists of epidermis and variable thickness of dermis.

Depending on the Depth of Dermal Involvement Skin Grafts are Classified into:

- Split thickness skin grafts (STSG) (Fig. 15.2).
- Full thickness skin grafts (FTSG) (Fig. 15.3).

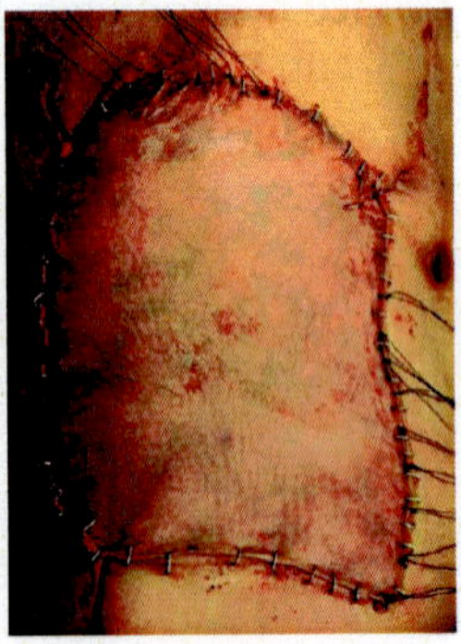

Fig. 15.2: Superficial thickness graft taken from abdomen

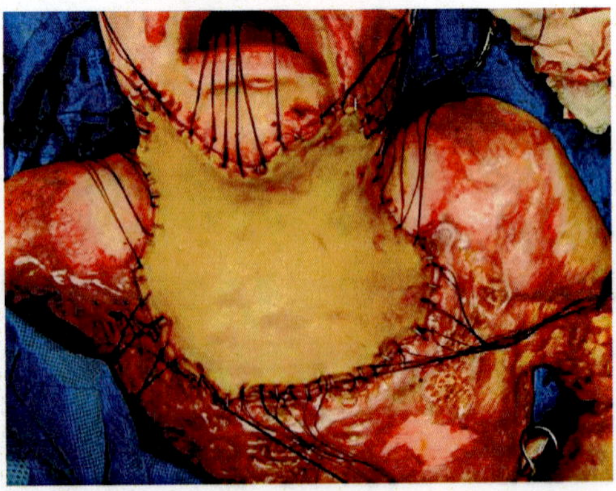

Fig.15.3: Full thickness skin graft to neck

Depending on the Donor (Species)

- Autografts- Skin is taken from the same individual from one area to the other area.
- Allograft- (homograft)- When skin is taken from one individual to another individual of the same species.
  - Example - skin from relatives (Fig. 15.4).

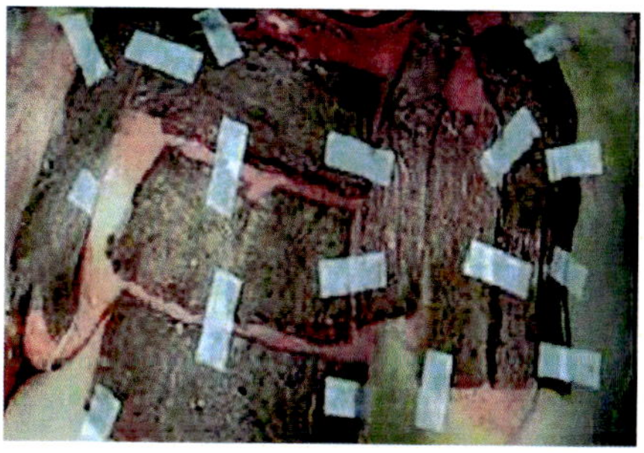

Fig. 15.4: Allograft (Homograft)

- Xenograft-(heterograft) when the skin is taken from one species to another species.
  - Example-from pig to human being.
- Isograft- when skin is transferred between identical twins.

15.3 INDICATION OF SKIN GRAFT

Skin graft is done to resurface raw areas.

15.4 CONTRAINDICATION OF SKIN GRAFT

Avascular Area

Areas which do not have good supply is contraindicated because skin graft does not have its own blood supply and have to depend on recipient site for its survival, hence graft will not take on bare bone, bare cartilage and bare tendon.

Infection

Absolute contraindication is beta hemolytic streptococcus, because streptococcus produces an enzyme called streptolysin which lysis or dissolves the fibrin bonds which is needed for the first stage of graft take.

Unhealthy Granulation Tissue

When the wound bed has slimy, pale tissue with copious discharge.

15.5 TAKE OF THE GRAFT

"Take of the graft" is a process when the grafted skin is firmly attached to the recipient site or when the graft has been vascularized. Graft can be sheet grafts or meshed grafts (Figs 15.5 and 15.6).

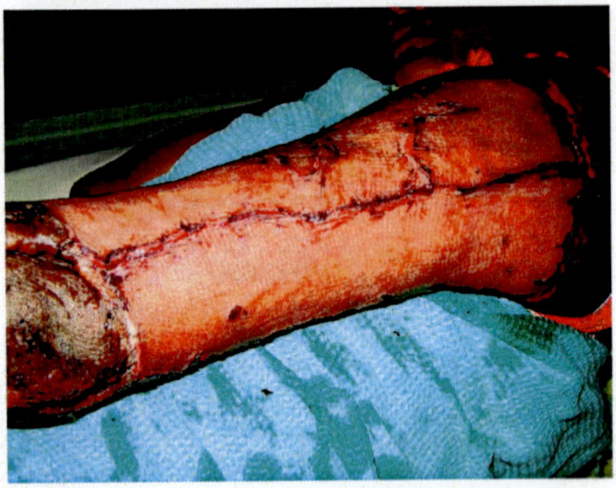

Fig. 15.5: Sheet graft

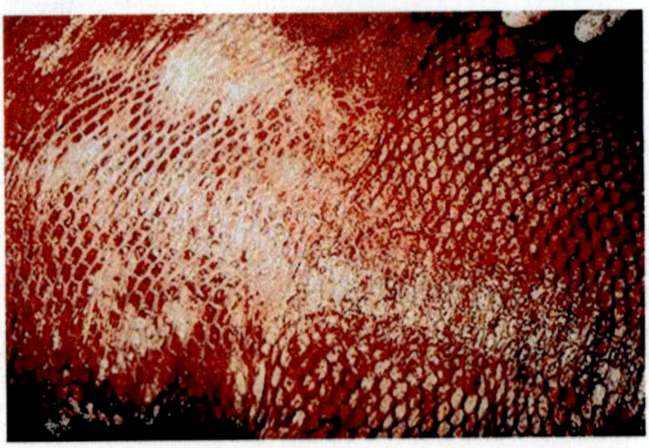

Fig. 15.6: Graft meshed using mesher

The Stages of Graft Take

- Plasmatic imbibition.
- Inosculation.
- Neovascularization.

Plasmatic Imbibition

For the first 24 hours after the graft has been applied. The graft derives its nutrition from the plasmatic serum which starts oozing from the raw area or bed. The graft imbibes this fluid. At the same time the fibrin network is also formed between the graft and the recipient site to hold the graft in place.

Inosculation

This means mouth to mouth contact of the blood vessels between the recipient bed and the graft to establish circulation.

Neovascularization

Many new blood vessels are formed between the graft and the bed leading to complete vascularization of the graft by 4th -5th day after graft application.

15.6 STORAGE OF SKIN GRAFT

Graft is stored at 4 degree centigrade in the refrigerator for about 21 days.

It can be stored in liquid nitrogen (-196 degree centigrade) over a longer period of time with out loss of viability.

15.7 POSTOPERATIVE CARE

Recipient Area

Secondary Wound

If the graft is applied on an infected wound or on an already existing wound, the graft should be inspected as early as possible so that even if pus is present it can be drained and the graft salvaged . After the first dressing the graft dressing should be done every day with moist dressing using either saline or betadine (The reason for moist dressing is that as long as the dressing is moist due to capillary action the pus gets absorbed from the bed) (Figs 15.7 to 15.9).

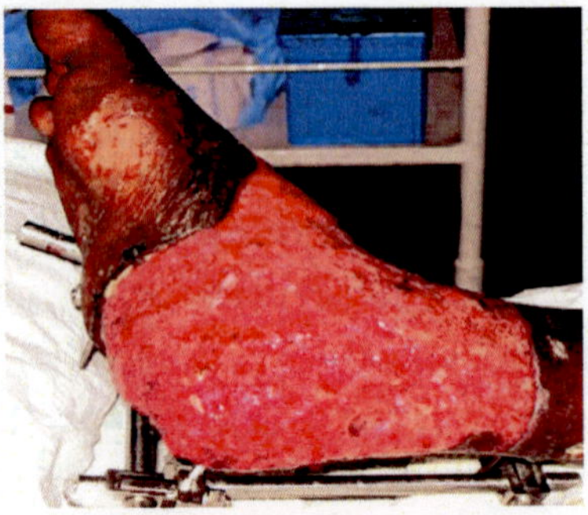

Fig. 15.7: Secondary wound

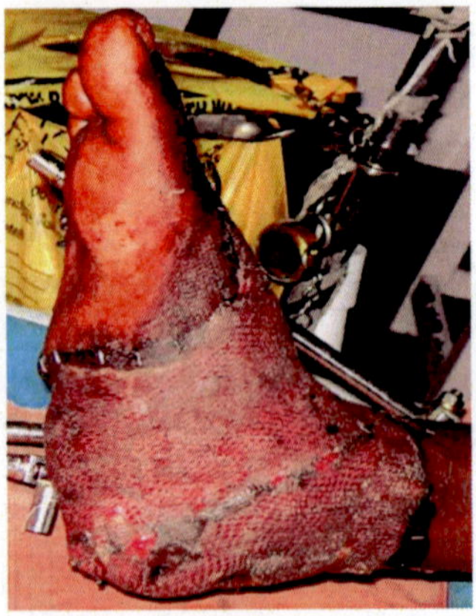

Fig. 15.8: Graft laid on secondary wound

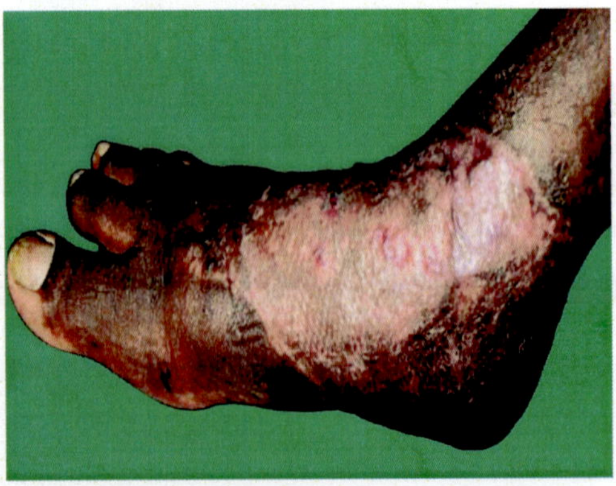

Fig. 15.9: Three months follow up

Primary Wound

Primary wound is one which is created on the operating table and is a clean wound, such wounds when grafted can be inspected after 10 days with out any fear of it being infected (Figs 15.10 to 5.12).

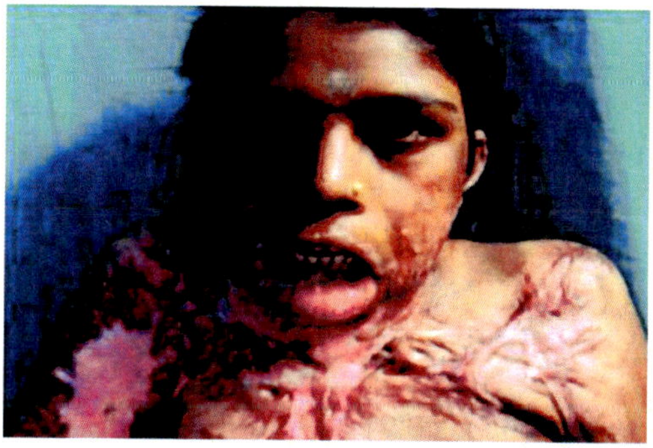

Fig. 15.10: Contracture neck

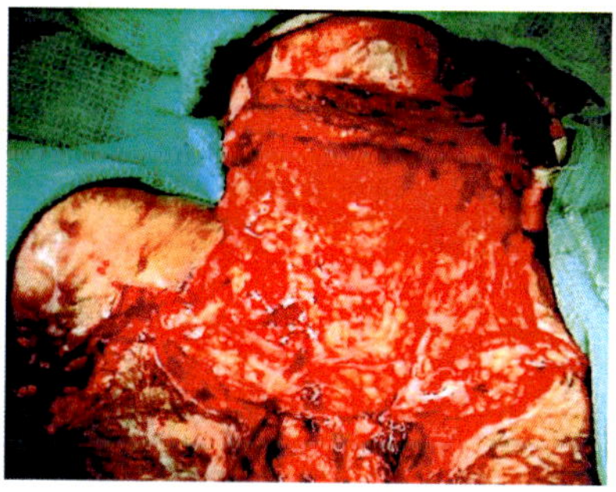

Fig. 15.11: Primary wound created on the table

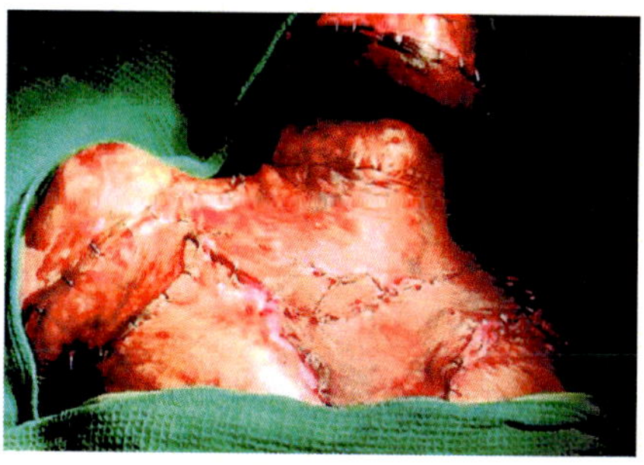

Fig. 15.12: Graft laid on primary wound

All grafted area have to be immobilized using plaster of paris splints for 10-days till the graft takes well and later should be replaced with alkathene splints for 6-8 months.

Donor Area

Method of Graft Harvesting (Figs 15.13 to 5.17).

Patients complain of severe pain in the donor area, this is because the nerve endings are exposed.

A lot of soakage is seen immediately after surgery and this requires only additional padding and bandage.

Elevation of grafted site using pillows is important to provide comfort to the patient.

Usually the donor site dressing should be removed by 10-14 days after surgery. If the dressing is adherent then soak the dressing with saline and gently remove without destroying the new epithelium. If there is infection then the dressing should be inspected early.

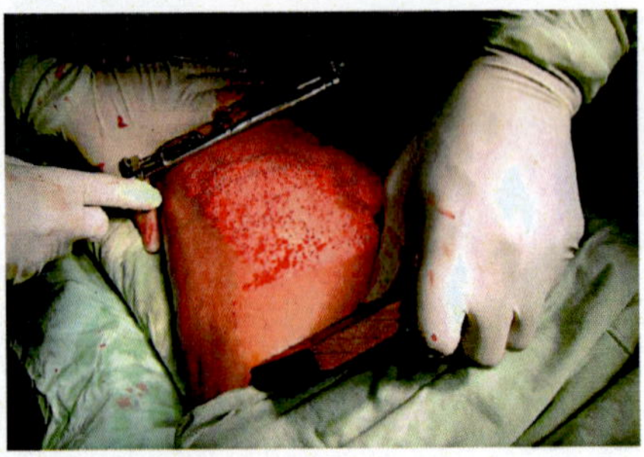

Fig. 15.13: Technique of taking skin graft by Humby's knife

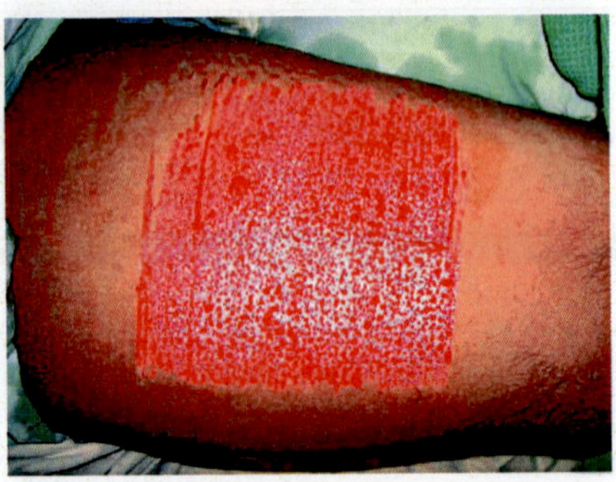

Fig. 15.14: Punctate bleeding seen in split thickness skin graft

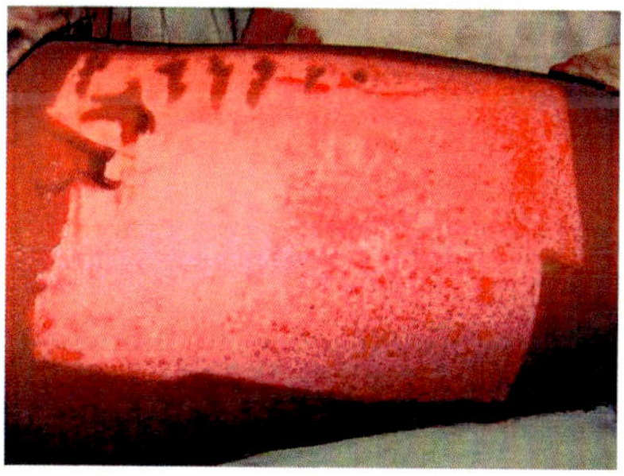

Fig. 15.15: Donor site bleeding controlled with adrenaline soaked gauze

Instrument Used

Some graft harvesting instruments are shown in Figs 15.16 to 15.18.

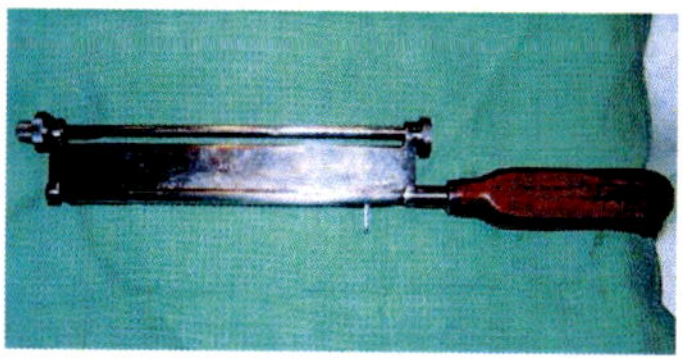

Fig. 15.16: Graft harvesting knife-Humby's

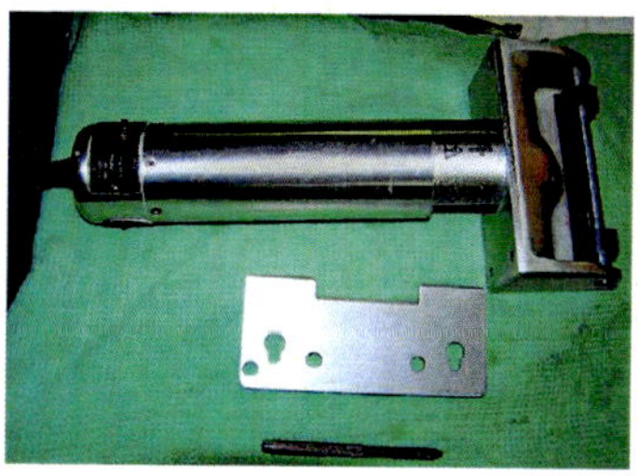

Fig. 15.17: Electric dermatome for graft taking

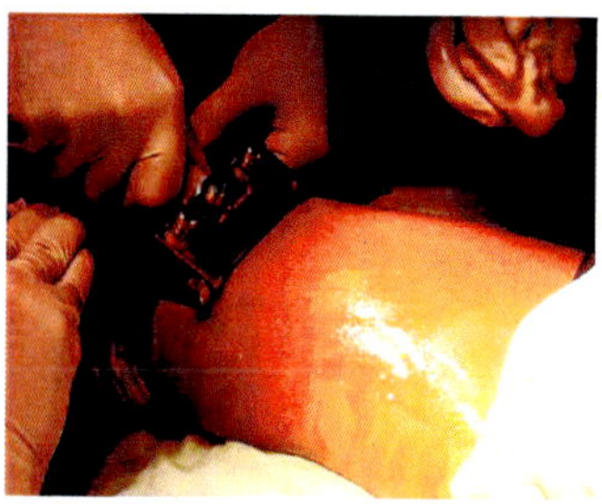

Fig. 15.18: Davis electric dermatome

Healing of Donor Site

Donor site heals spontaneously in 10-15 days by epithelialization from the epidermal structures like the hair follicle, sweat glands and the sebaceous glands which are present in the dermis (these are epidermal structures but invade dermis to variable extent). Different skin substitutes are used to reduce pain and to hasten skin graft take (Figs 15.19 to 15.32).

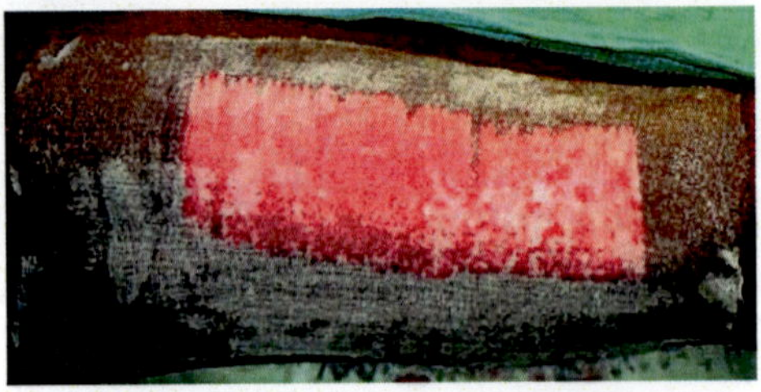

Fig. 15.19: Donor dressing with paraffin gauze

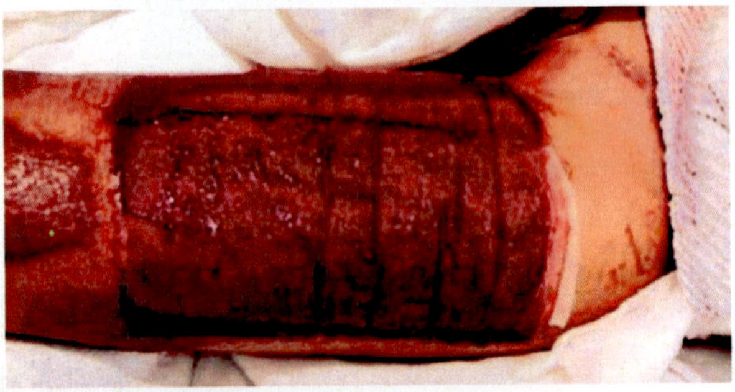

Fig. 15.20: Donor dressing with scarlet red gauze

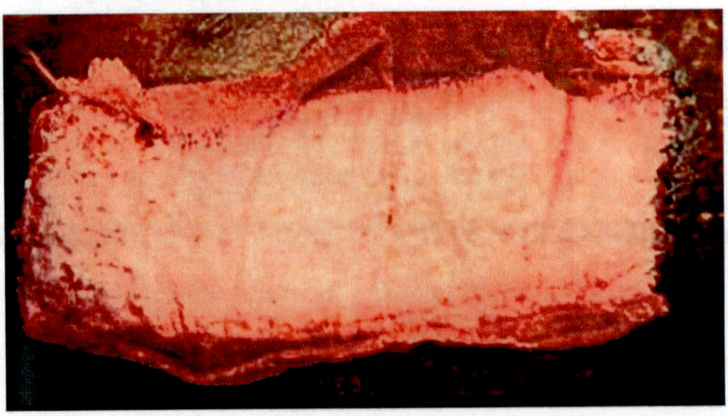

Fig. 15.21: Donor dressing dry and adherent

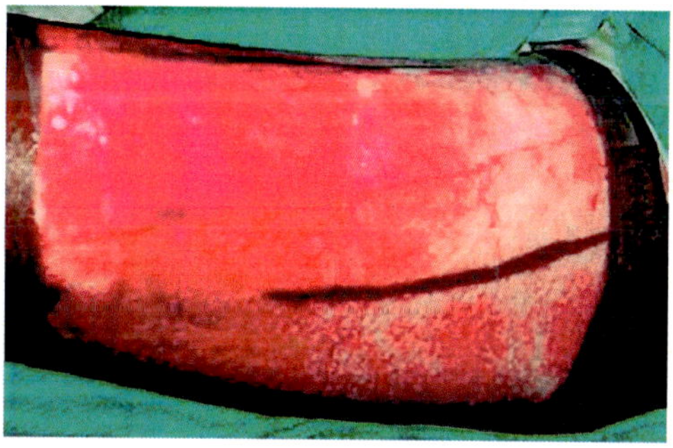

Fig. 15.22: Healicoll sheet for donor area

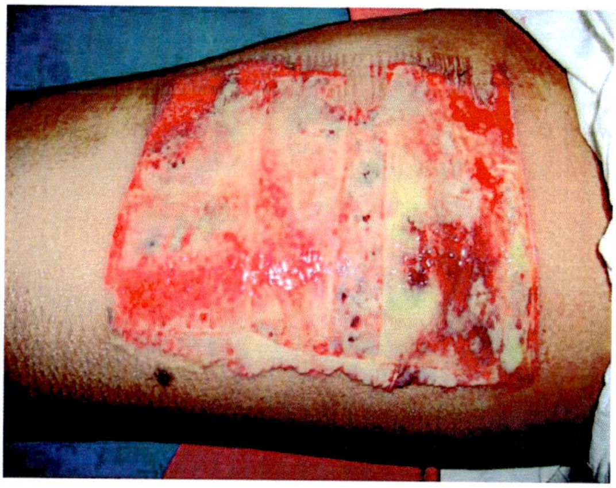

Fig. 15.23: Donor site after 5 days of healicoll application

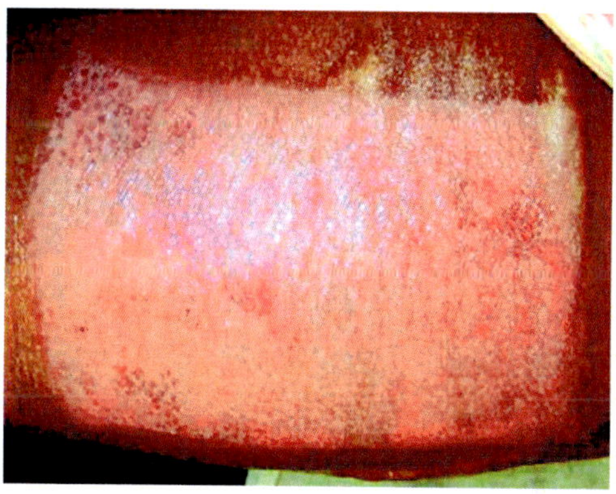

Fig. 15.24: Donor site healed

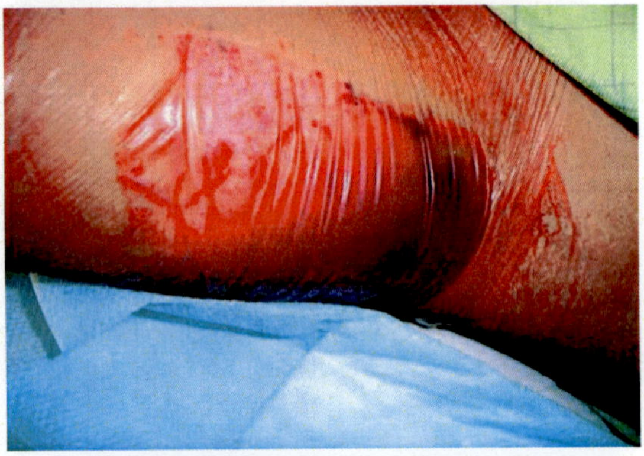

Fig. 15.25: Opsite for donor site

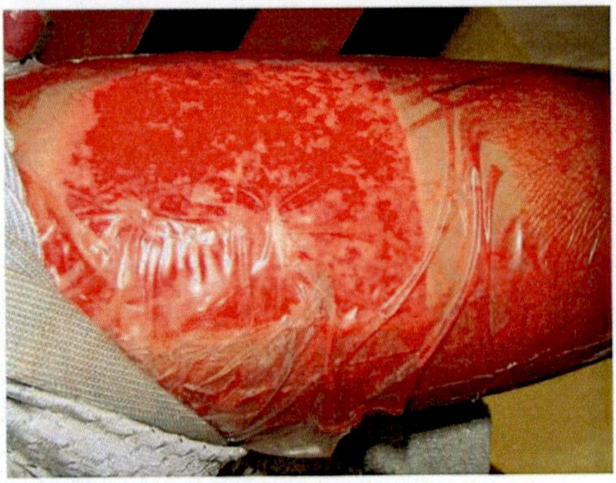

Fig. 15.26: Maceration seen under opsite dressing

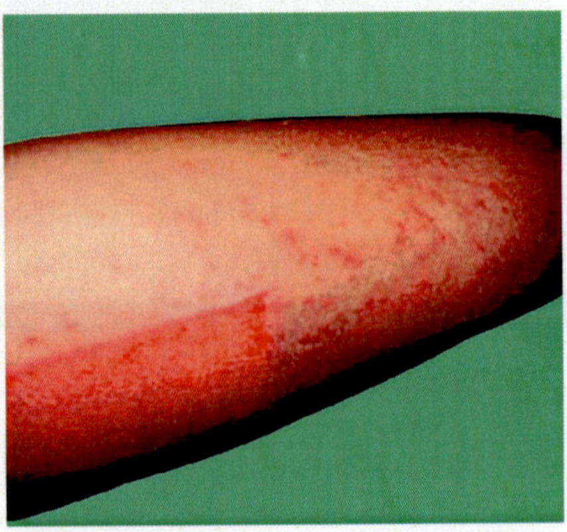

Fig. 15.27: Rashes in opsite used areas

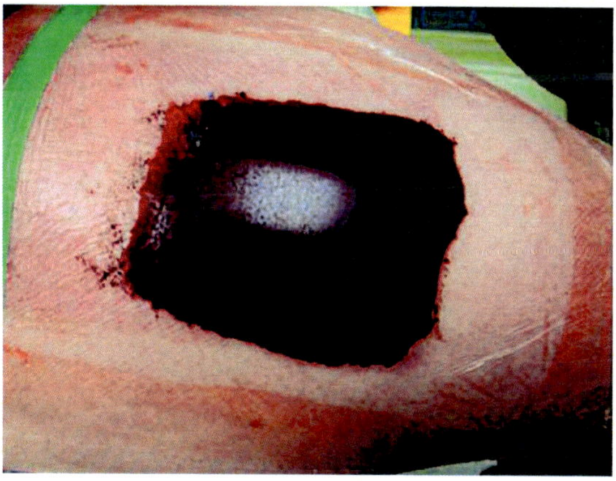

Fig. 15.28: Blood collection under opsite

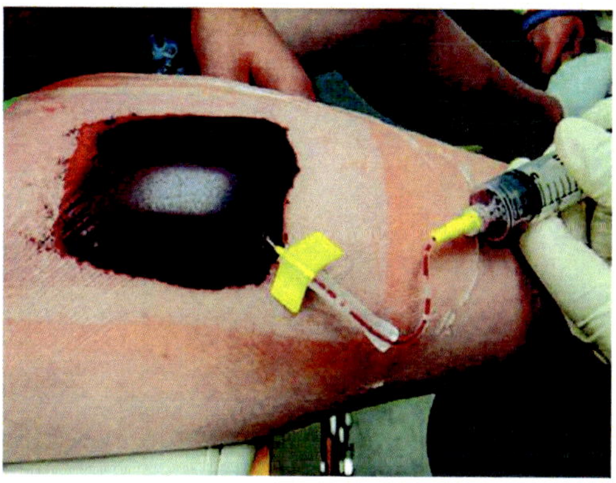

Fig. 15.029: Aspiration of blood

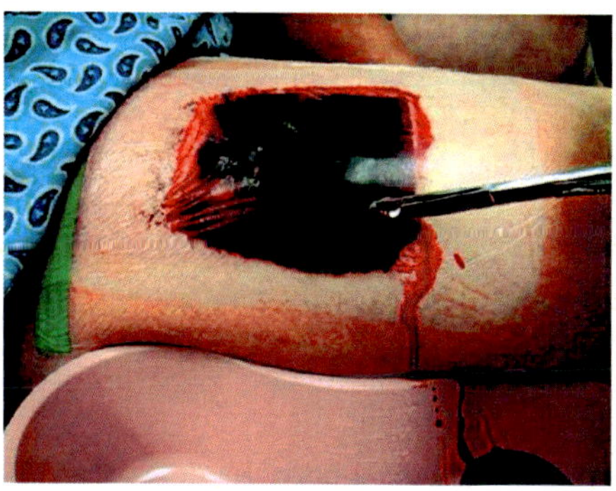

Fig. 15.30: Nick in the opsite to remove blood collection

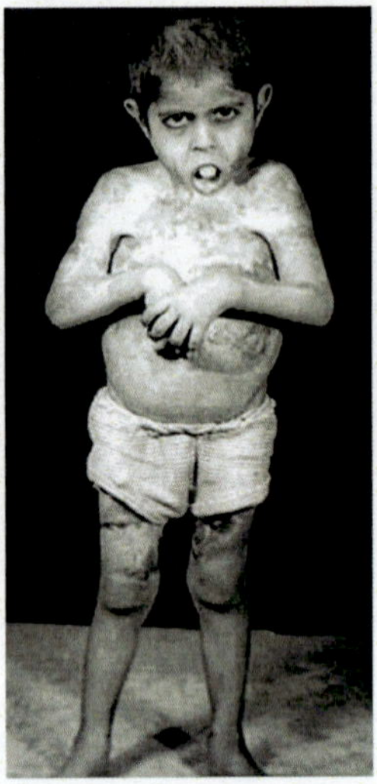

Fig. 15.31: Severe contracture

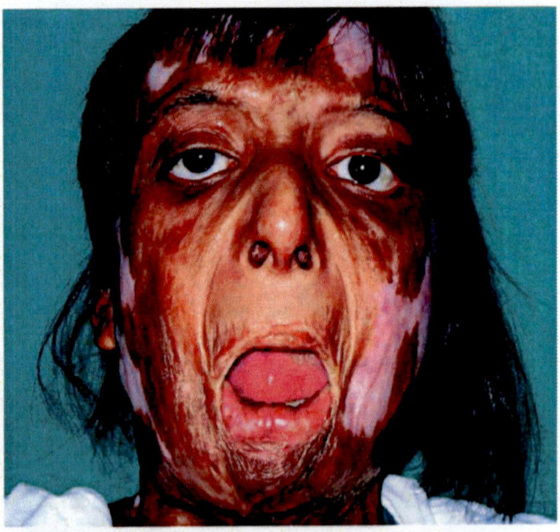

Fig. 15.32: Pigmentation changes

15.8 PHYSICAL CHANGES IN THE SKIN GRAFT

Graft Contraction

Once the graft is applied it starts showing contraction due to the myofibroblasts in the recipient blood. This contraction starts after

10 days and continues for a year. It is thus very important to prevent this contracture by applying pressure garments, splints and moisturizing lotion for atleast a year.

Split thickness grafts are usually dry and for it to have a normal texture moisturizing creams and lotions have to be applied as early as 10th postoperative day atleast 5 times a day and continued for 6- 8 months.

Pigment Changes

Generally graft tends to become darker. Various methods to prevent hyperpigmentation are:

- To avoid sunlight
- Use of sun protecting factor > 15 % (fair and lovely cream)
- Use of sun shade caps/umbrella
- Bleaching creams
- Dermabrasion

Sun Blocking Agent

Direct effects of sunlight has both acute and chronic changes on the skin :

- Acute changes are - Sunburn and tanning
- Chronic changes are - Premature aging
  - Premalignant skin lesion
  - Malignant skin lesion.

A sunscreen is a photoprotective agent designed to reduce the effects of UV radiation from the sun. It acts by absorption, reflection or scattering of solar rays. Upon application sunscreens act as filters and inhibit the penetration of UV rays to the cells of epidermis and dermis and thereby reduce pigmentation changes. The other photoprotecting measures are clothing and sun avoidance. A commonly used sun screen is para amino benzoic acid (PABA). The most common measure of sunscreen effectiveness is a sun protecting factor (SPF) of 15 or greater. Sun screen should be applied 15-30 minutes before actual solar exposure.

15.9 ROLE OF NURSE IN SKIN GRAFT CARE

Preoperative Care

- Patient should be prepared mentally preoperatively about the post op pain and care.
- The donor area should be washed with soap and water, shaved and prepared with spirit.
- A sterile towel is wrapped around the prepared area before sending the patient to the operation theater.

Postoperative Care

Day-1

- After the surgery the part is elevated to minimize the edema.
- Donor area is observed for excessive oozing . If there is bleeding add additional pads and bandage.

Day-1-9

- Recipient site -If there is no infection, the first dressing is done on the 9th postoperative day.

  Steps that a nurse should take to help the doctor in removing the dressing is

  1. Wash your hand.
  2. Keep a mackintosh under the dressing site.
  3. Wear clean gloves and remove the outer dressing.
  4. Soak the dressing by pouring normal saline for 10 minutes.
  5. This will help the doctor to remove the dressing easily with out harming the graft or causing pain to the patient.
  6. Cut the excess dry graft.
  7. If there is any collection press the graft gently with a moist gauze.
  8. Finally clean the wound and dress with liquid paraffin.
- Liquid paraffin dressings are continued from day 9-15.
- Subsequently moisturizing cream and massage is advised 5 times/day followed by splinting, pressure garment and silicone gel.

Donor Site

If there is no donor site infection, the dressing is gently removed up to the gauze layer without injuring the new epithelium on the 10th day and the wound is inspected before the patient leaves the ward.

- If the wound has healed well, advice liquid paraffin application or coconut oil application daily atleast 3-5 times a day.
- If there are signs of hypertrophy advice pressure garment.

Chapter

16 SKIN SUBSTITUTES

16.1 INTRODUCTION

- Skin substitutes for temporary covering has become a more frequent requirement.
- The extensive burns leave behind so few available donor sites that their wounds cannot be covered by autografts, hence skin substitutes have become more important.
- Early wound closure with minimal or no scarring is the ultimate aim in management of extensive burns. Superficial burns are the burns which heal by epithelialization and deep burns require skin cover for wound closure. In extensive burns there is paucity of donor area. The wound needs to be covered temporarily till we harvest or procure autograft. As the name implies skin substitutes are the material used to cover the wound.

16.2 CLASSIFICATION

Temporary

A. **Biological:** Amniotic membrane, homograft, collagen.

B. **Synthetic:** Biobrane, transcyte, opsite.

Semi-Permanent

A. Dermal replacement (biological) with epidermal substitutes (Synthetic) : Integra.

B. Synthetic dermal matrix only: Dermagraft.

Permanent

A. *Dermal replacement:* Alloderm, healicoll.

B. *Epidermal replacement:* Cultured keratinocyte.

C. *Composite dermal and epidermal replacement:* Dermal epidermal cultured graft.

16.3 ADVANTAGES OF SKIN SUBSTITUTES

- Hastens wound maturation.
- Maintains microbial control.
- Normalization of blood proteins and hematocrit levels.
- Protects the wound.
- Reduction of water, protein and electrolyte losses.
- Reduction of heat dispersion.
- Reduces pain.

16.4 PROPERTIES OF SKIN SUBSTITUTES

- Adherence.
- Absence of antigenicity.
- Absence of local and systemic toxicity.
- Biodegradability.
- Compatibility.
- Elasticity to permit motion of underlying tissue.
- Flexibility and pliability.
- Impermeable to exogenous microorganism.
- Rapid adherence to wound surface.
- Resistance to shear stress.

16.5 TYPES OF SKIN SUBSTITUTES

Biological

- Homograft.
- Heterograft-Pigskin.
- Amniotic membrane.
- Collagen-Healicoll.

Synthetic

- Opsite.
- Omiderm.

Biosynthetic

- Biobrane.
- Transcyte.
- Integra.

Collagen based dermal analog

- Deepithelialized allograft.

Culture derived tissue

- Cultured autologous keratinocytes.

Biological

Allograft (Homograft)

- Cadaver allograft provides temporary cover for extensive burns.
- Used as a temporary burn dressing for full thickness burns.
- Immediate coverage for superficial burns.
- Used as a test to determine the likelihood of autograft take.
- Recent improvements in immunosuppression therapy gives some promise for permanent skin allografting to succeed.

Advantages

- Reduction in water, electrolyte and protein loss.
- Reduction in wound infection rates.
- Reduction in pain.

Disadvantages

- Need for refrigerated storage conditions.
- A limited effective shelf life of 7-10 days at 4 degree.
- Viability and take decrease with time.
- Possibility of disease transmission is high.

Frozen Skin

Advantages

- Maintains viability
- Can adhere to the wounds, viable and able to take and stimulate vascularization.
- Showed to be less antigenic than fresh skin and this permits a lasting take.

Disadvantages

- Requires the creation of an expensive and complex organizational operative and legislative system.
- Fear of transmission of AIDS.

Heterografts (xenografts)

- Skin from various animals including, pig, frog, and sheep are harvested . This is processed in a number of ways to reduce the antigenicity and prolong adherence. Porcine xenografts can confer many of the same advantages as allograft skin. They effectively retard evaporative water loss, reduce infection and encourage autologous epidermal growth. When applied to wounds it will adhere but not vascularize, making it most useful as a temporary covering.
- Bovine and porcine skin harvested and stored are used extensively in burns.
- Porcine skin resembles human skin and hence it is the most commonly used heterograft.

Advantages

- Used as temporary burn dressing.
- Also available as a biosynthetic dressing off the shelf as E-Z DERM.
- Has all the properties of skin and it encourages re-epithelialization.

Disadvantages

- A lab set up is required for processing.
- Not so effective in reducing bacterial population.
- Adherence to wound bed is less.
- Inosculation does not take place.
- It undergoes progressive necrosis.
- Strict immobilization is necessary.

Amniotic Membrane (Davis 1910)

- It is the inner layer of tissue that surrounds the fetus *in utero* and contains amniotic fluid . Both the inner amnion and the outer chorion have been used as skin substitutes.
- Amnion is preferred as it is less antigenic. It contains substantial amounts of many growth factors that stimulate epithelial

proliferation but also has antiangiogenic qualities. The use of amniotic membranes was questioned after risks of disease transmission became widely recognized.

- Amnion exerts an angiogenic effect, which increases capillary density of the wound bed.
- It enhances epithelialization in partial thickness burns and promotes epithelial ingrowths from wound margins in full thickness burn wounds.

Advantages

- It is easy, simple and inexpensive, prevents heat and fluid loss.
- Set up required is simple.
- Easy to apply, readily available, provides pain relief.
- Can be used for all superficial burns where it promotes healing.
- Adheres well and peels off spontaneously.
- Has an angiogenic effect and increases capillary density.
- Long term glycerol preserved amniotic membrane is available.

Disadvantage - Cross infection is common and dangerous

Indication - Fresh burns
Superficial second degree burns

Requirments - For storage
100 ml normal saline
Injection crystalline penicillin 10 L
Injection Gentamycin 80 mg.

16.6 HEALICOLL: (NEW PRODUCT WITH EXCITING EXPERIENCE)

- Healicoll is a type-1 pure collagen membrane derived from bovine source and maintains a moist environment at the wound surface and is biocompatible, biologically active, biodegradable and bioengineered skin substitute with absence of antigenecity, low cost, long shelf life and minimum storage requirements. It accelerates the healing process and improves the quality of the wound. It gets totally absorbed, there is no itching, no irritation, no impairment to movement, no further nursing care required, hospitalization and cost are significantly reduced. It is stored at room temp with a shelf life of 3 years.

- Accelerated healing is due to epithelial cells migration towards the clot and allows it to be reorganized, induces platelet aggregation and provide hemostasis. The inflammatory cells like the neutrophils and macrophages invade the clot and secrete growth factors that attract fibroblasts for repair.
- Effectiveness of healicoll is attributed to the bioengineered feature of the pure type-1 collagen. The uncrossed healicoll has improved cell signalling to produce molecule for repair and regeneration.
- It is useful as a donor site dressing material, and in superficial thickness skin defects.
- It is helps to accelerate the rate of epithelialization.
- It significantly reduces post-operative pain.
- Healicoll treatment significantly reduces the operation time, hospital stay and cost of treatment.
- Healicoll is consistently shown to form a clear gel like layer of tissue on 5th post application day in all cases and ready to support take of skin graft.
- The results show the effects of healicoll healing in exposed bones joints and tendons.
- Healicoll treatment provides high quality, efficacious, efficient and cost effective wound care.

Methods

Application procedure (Figs 16.1 to 16.8)

Healicoll collagen comes in a sterile pack. The collagen sheet is covered by a transparent film on one side and by an opaque plastic backing sheet on the other. The pack is soaked in sterile water for 3-5 minutes, the outer transparent sheet is peeled off. It is then applied over the area to be covered along with the backing sheet for easy handling. The white backing sheet is removed and the transparent pliable helicoll sheet is applied on the wound, making sure that all air bubbles are removed. Apply paraffin gauze impregnated with antibiotic and bandage. Healicoll dressing was applied once only unless the dressing got relocated and removed from the site of application.

Dressing

During pilot study wound was inspected every day to see the changes. Our finding on the 5th post healicoll application day was interesting . Healicoll undergoes degradation on day 5 and the shiny healicoll is completely absent and in its place a gel like substance is present which gets incorporated in the wound from day 5.

Healicoll can be used successfully for reconstruction of complex wounds obviating the need for flap cover . This method has minimal patient morbidity, and hospital stay and has proved a successful modality for healing wounds that otherwise have been difficult to heal and may offer best option for definitive management of extensive full thickness defects. Healicoll promotes wound healing, and has potential as a dermal substitute.

Its availability at a low cost in India and potential applicability in a wide range of clinical scenarios offers enormous advantages.

It is suitable in pediatric and adult patients. It is safe, effective dressing for reduction of infection , increases reepithelization, less change of dressing, thus cost effective dressing for burns. The bioengineered tissue could be rapidly vascularized by inosculation with the host vessels and the skin equivalent become a permanent skin replacement.

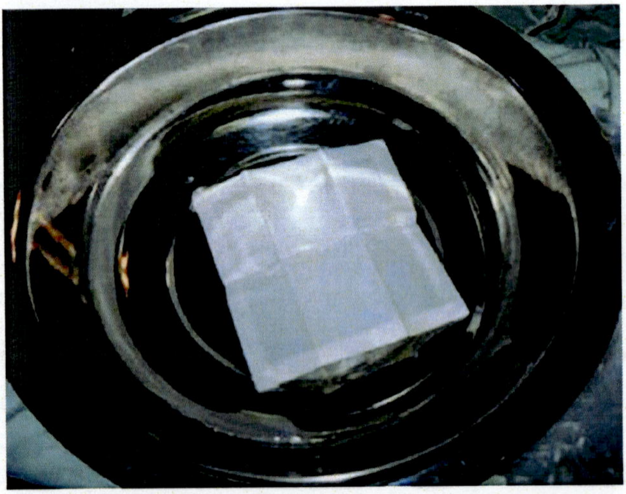

Fig. 16.1: Healicoll soaking in sterile water before application

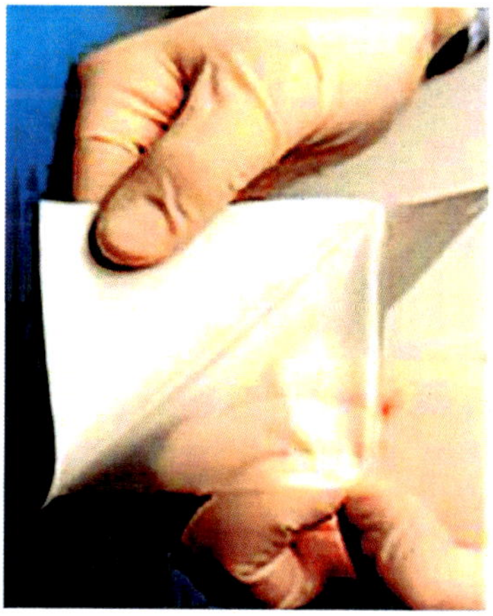

Fig. 16.2: Healicoll outer layer being peeled

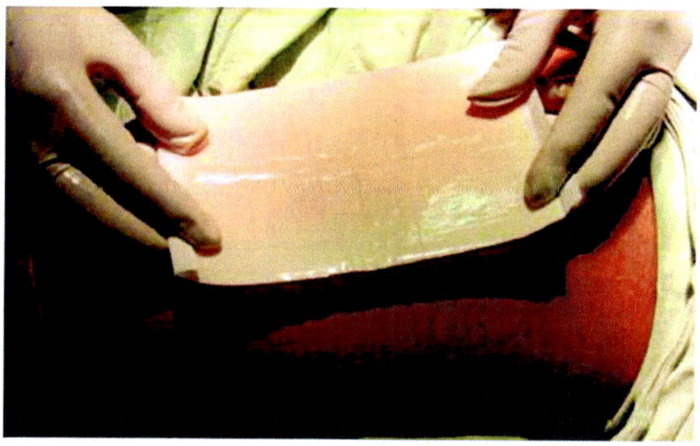

Fig. 16.3: Healicoll applied over the wound with backing sheet

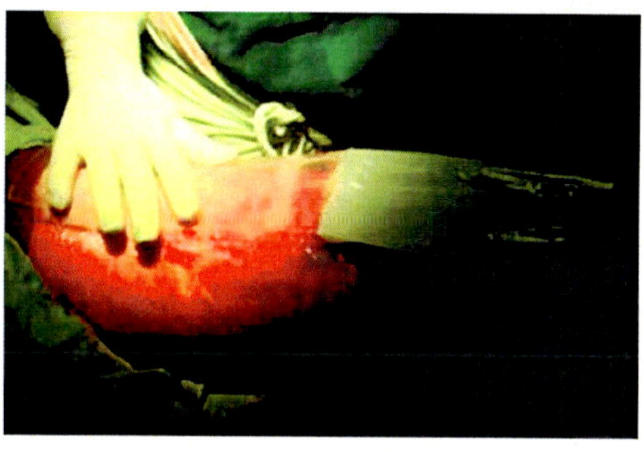

Fig. 16.4: Healicoll backing sheet removed

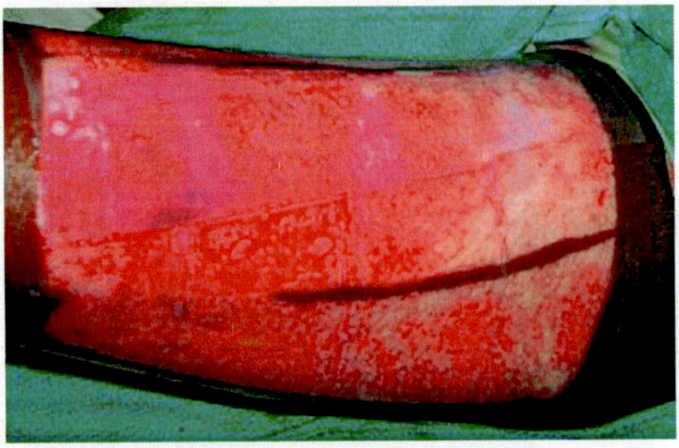

Fig. 16.5: Healicoll sheet in situ with all air bubbles removed

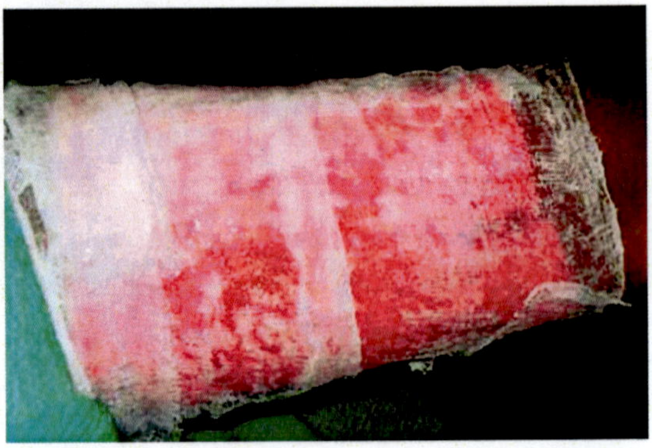

Fig. 16.6: Healicoll covered with paraffin gauze

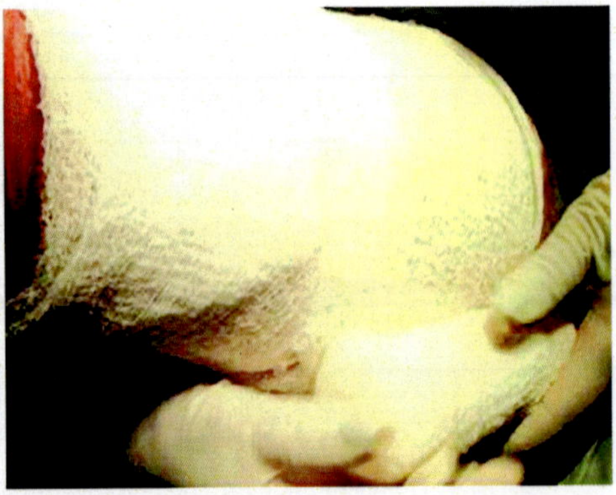

Fig. 16.7: Healicoll covered with bandage

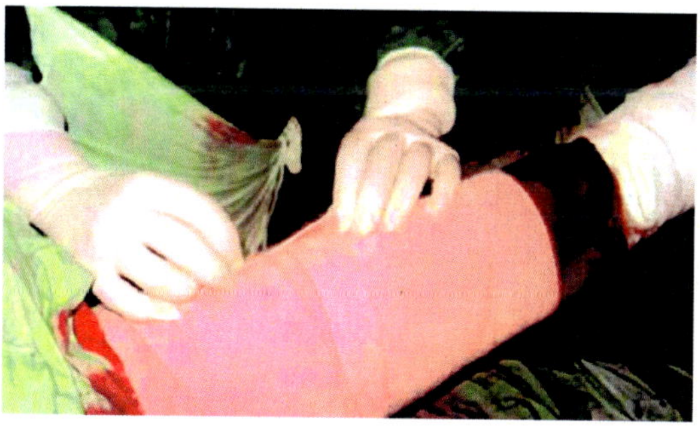

Fig. 16.8: Apply elastocrepe bandage

16.7 SYNTHETIC SKIN SUBSTITUTES (FIG. 16.9)

Omiderm is a thin transparent polyurethane based membrane. It sticks to the moist wound surface. Its transparency facilitates easy observation of the burn wound.

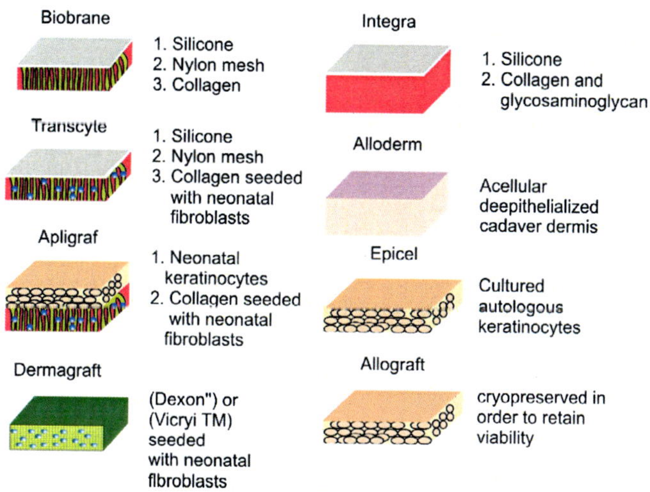

Fig. 16.9: Skin substitutes

Biosynthetic (Rational for Developing)

- Given the limitations of available biologic bilayer skin, the development of engineered skin substitutes become necessary using synthetic component.
- Incorporating biological active components such as collagen, glycosaminoglycan, keratinocytes and fibroblasts.

Chapter 17

PAIN MANAGEMENT

17.1 TYPES OF PAIN

- Continuous pain due to injuries.
- Acquired pain due to therapeutic procedures.

17.2 OBJECTIVES OF PAIN MANAGEMENT

- To minimize pain.
- To promote sense of caring and give them confidence.
- To reduce the stress of pain and thereby reduce hypermetabolism.
- To provide comfort.

17.3 CLINICAL VARIATION OF PAIN

- Varies from patient to patient.
- Continuous pain.
- Pain due to therapeutic procedures.
- Pain due to healing (itching).

17.4 ROUTES OF ADMINISTRATION

- Initially in the resuscitative period the absorption of drugs through intramuscular route is uncertain and hence all sedation and analgesic should be given by intravenous route.

Commonly Used Analgesics

- Injection morphine.
- Injection pethidine.

Side Effects

- Opiates like morphine cause nausea , respiratory depression and dependence.

17.5 TO OVER COME PROBLEMS

- Training in relaxation , distraction, audio and video and finally seeking chaplaincy department.

Chapter

18 OUT-PATIENT CARE

Advances in burn care have improved burn mortality and shortened hospital stay. This has enabled health care providers to treat more patients with burns as outpatients to reduce the cost of treatment.

The goals of an out-patient burn clinic should be

- To provide daily wound care.
- To educate patient.
- To prevent unnecessary admissions.
- To promote early discharge for hospitalized patients.
- Wound care should be provided by burn unit nurses because they often require the special expertise of burn unit nurses. This leads to better results and more consistent follow up. Patient satisfaction is increased and teaching the patient about wound care is provided by an experienced staff.

18.1 EXISTING METHOD

- Out patient burn care is generally held biweekly when patients attend the OPD services.
- Patient who require daily dressing care either go to emergency department for follow up or have to be admitted in the hospital.

Disadvantage of this Method

- Patient education regarding dressing care, signs and symptoms of complication and the anticipated wound healing process is often lacking.
- Lack of expertise in burn care results in more outpatient visits, more anxiety and stress for the patients and family.

How to Over Come

- Burn clinic should be established on the burn unit to provide a high standard of care.
- Provide daily wound care and teaching for out patients which prevents unnecessary admissions.
- Helps in planning for earlier discharge from hospital.

18.2 DESIGN OF THE BURN CLINIC

- Should be separate from the inpatient treatment facilities. This facilitates infection control.
- Separate burn nurses should be designated to provide outpatient wound care with out disrupting inpatient care 7 days a week.
- The next phase would be to train
  - Burn registrars.
  - Burn nurses.
  - Nurse anesthetist.

Implementation

- Patients are evaluated in the emergency department by a resident physician, assess burn wound and determine whether the patient requires hospitalization or outpatient treatment.
- If out patient treatment, doctor contacts the clinic nurse.
- On arrival patient is registered and taken to the dressing room for wound care.

18.3 WOUND CARE

- Wound cleaned thoroughly, all dead skin are removed, blisters are ruptured, once wound is clean, apply either biological skin cover or synthetic skin cover and allow it to dry for few hours.
- Instruction is given to the patient or relatives to take care of the wound.
- Regular follow up needed for supervision.

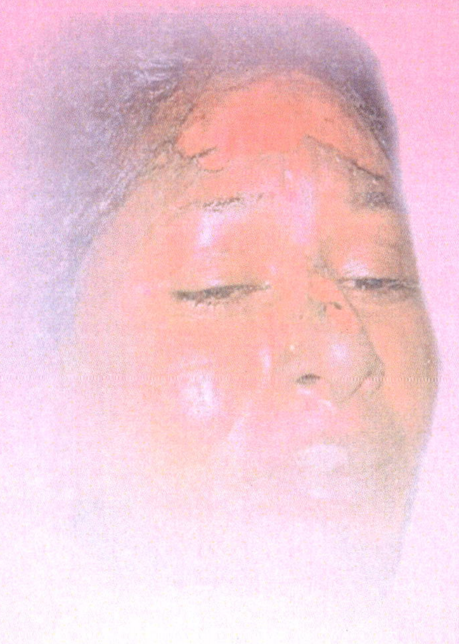

Section Three

COMPLICATIONS: EARLY AND LATE

Chapter 19 COMPLICATIONS ENCOUNTERED IN BURNS

19.1 IMMEDIATE

1. *Hypovolemic shock:* Due to fluid and electrolyte imbalance.
2. *Hemoconcentration:* Plasma is lost from the vascular compartment. resulting in only RBC being present in the compartment.
3. *Reduced urinary output:* Renal blood flow is reduced.
4. *Sodium loss:* Edema fluid shifts into the cell along with water sodium is also lost.
5. *Potassium excess:* Massive cellular trauma.
6. *Respiratory complication:* Inhalation injury.
7. Extensive circumferential burns on the chest causing constriction effect.

19.2 INTERMEDIATE

1. Wound infection (Figs 19.1 to 19.3).
2. ARDS
3. Septicemia.

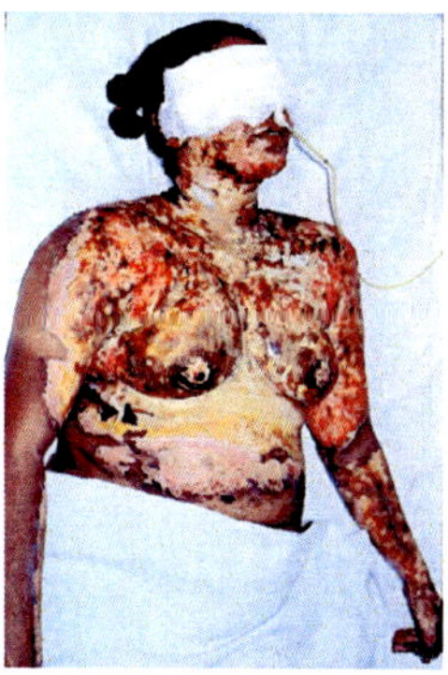

Fig. 19.1: Local signs of sepsis

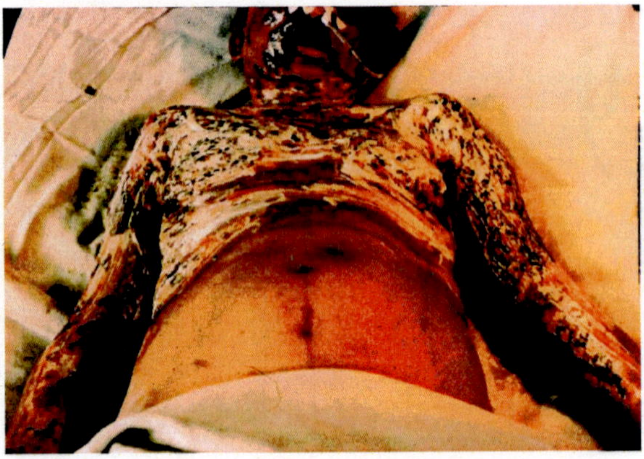

Fig. 19.2: Severe local infection

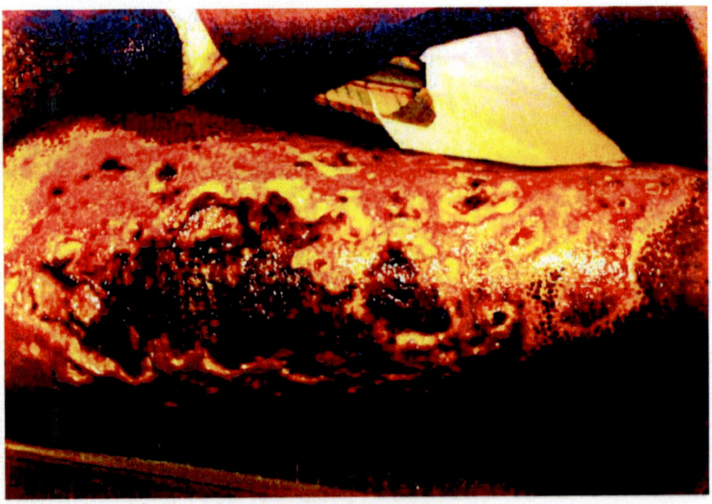

Fig. 19.3: Local infection

19.3 LATE

1. Contracture (Figs 19.4 to 19.9) .
2. Hypertrophic scars and pigmentation changes (Figs 19.10 and 19.11).
3. Hand and foot deformities (Figs 19.12 and 19.13).

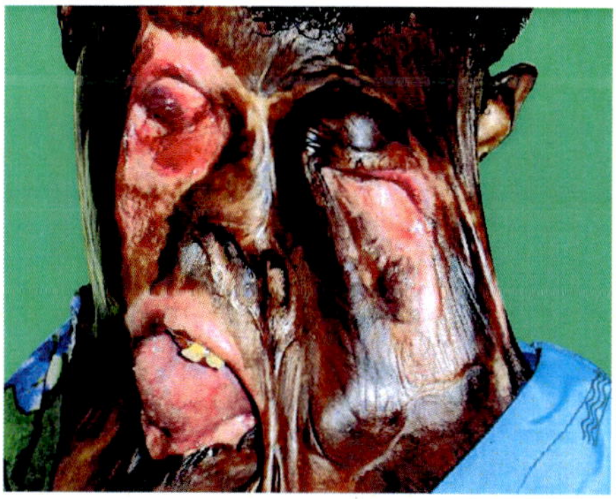

Fig. 19.4: Severe contracture

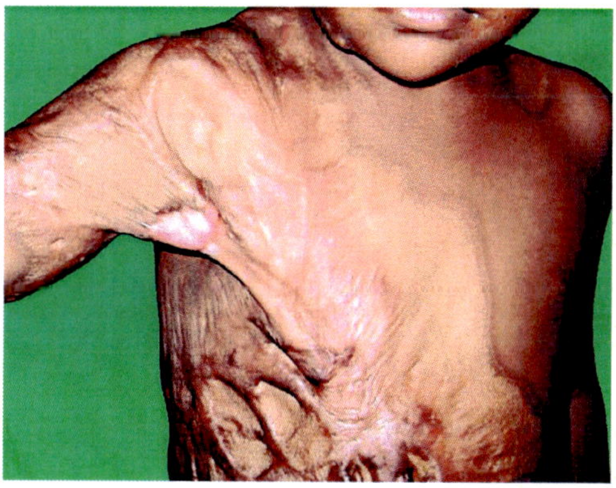

Fig. 19.5: Axillary contracture

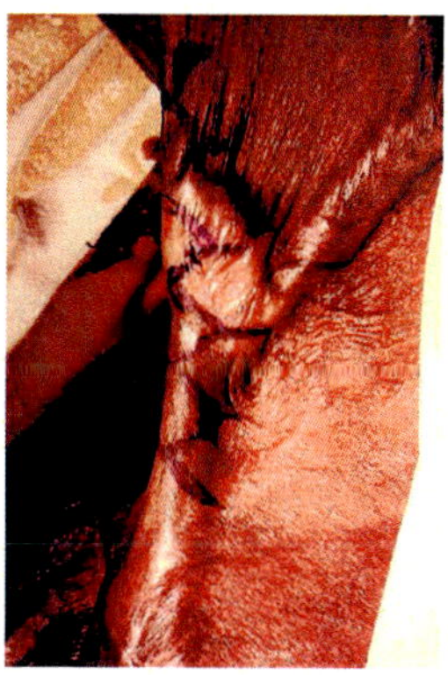

Fig. 19.6: Axillary contracture released by multiple V-Y flap

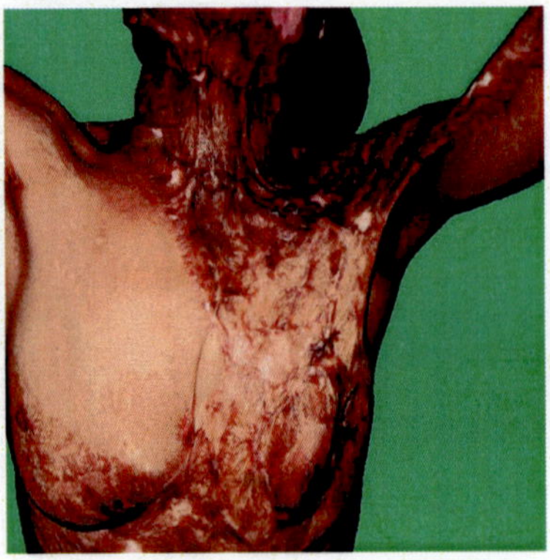

Fig. 19.7: Axillary and breast contracture

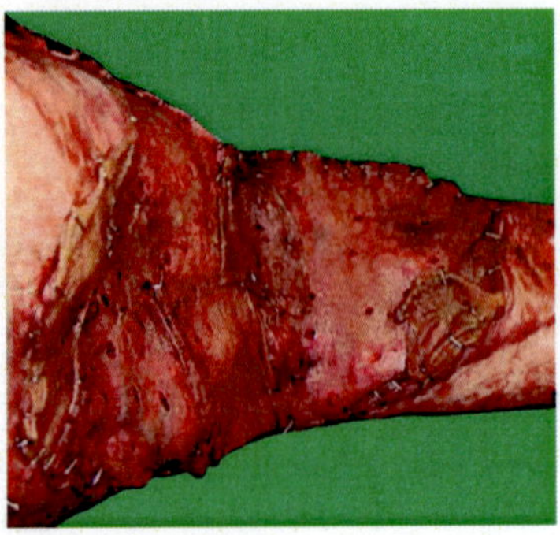

Fig. 19.8: Axillary contracture treated with skin graft

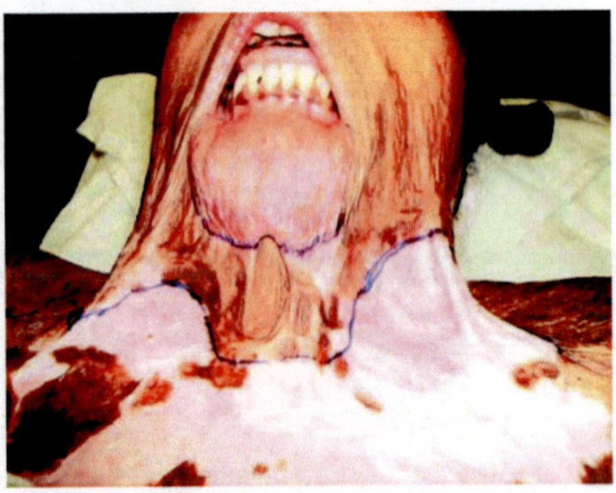

Fig. 19.9: Severe contracture of lip

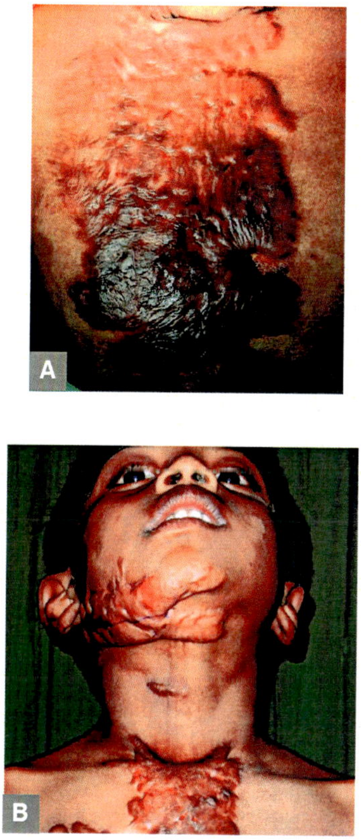

Figs 19.10 A and B: Hypertrophic scars

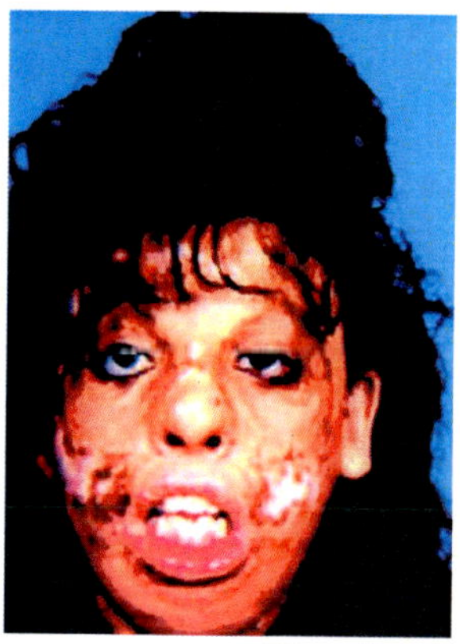

Fig. 19.11: Pigmentation changes

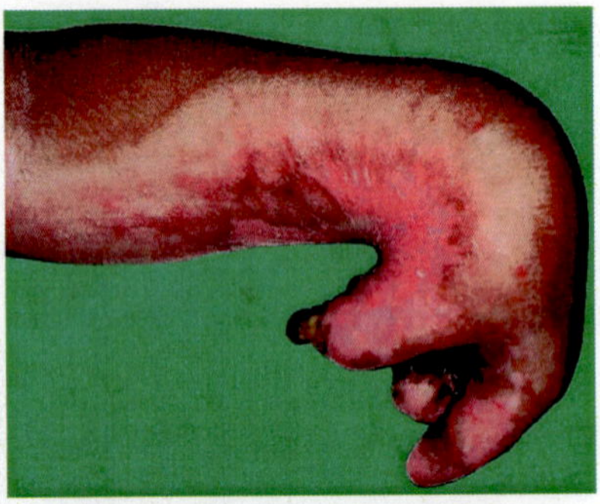

Fig. 19.12: Severe hand deformity

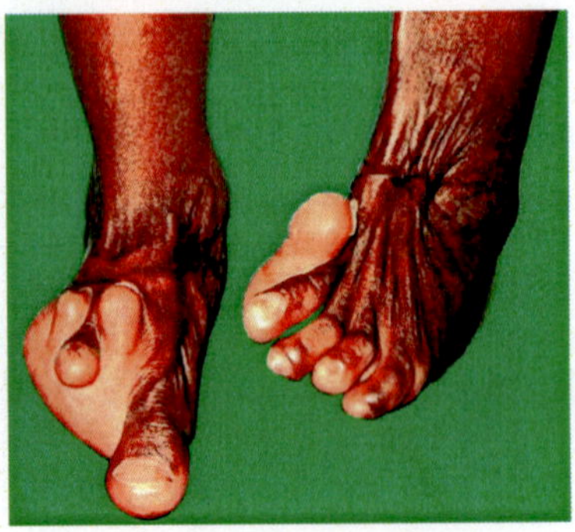

Fig. 19.13: Foot deformity

Chapter 20

BURN WOUND SEPSIS

- Wound infection generally occurs when the bacterial count is greater than 10^5 per gram of tissue.
- Whether the infection remains localized to the wound, spreads to the adjacent tissues, or becomes systemic depends on the interaction of the invading microbes and the host defenses.
- Human skin contains many organisms in which the individual co-exists and equilibrium is established.
- In burn patients this equilibrium is disturbed and sepsis occurs.

20.1 FACTORS RESPONSIBLE FOR BURN WOUND INFECTION

1. Poor general health.
2. Weak defences of the burn victim.
3. Fertile culture medium offered by dead burned tissue.
4. Presence of pathogenic bacteria.

20.2 CLASSIFICATION OF BURN WOUND

Colonization

Micro-organisms are present in the necrotic tissue of the burn wound, contaminated from the environment.

Septic Burn Wound

It is also known as invasive wound infection. Here the micro organisms invade viable tissue, but infection is only localized.

Burn Wound Sepsis

Micro organisms invade viable tissue along with systemic spread through blood and lymphatic channels. The first systemic signs of sepsis is a rising respiratory rate.

Septicemia (Sepsis)

Proliferation of bacteria in the bloodstream.

Septic Shock

Septic shock is a term used to describe the combination of septicemia and shock.

It is also called endotoxic shock because the endotoxin released from the gram negative bacilli is responsible for the widespread intravascular damage.

20.3 VARIOUS FACTORS RESPONSIBLE FOR BURN WOUND CONTAMINATION

- The method of contamination can be either direct transfer of bacteria to the wound or through bloodstream.
- The various source of infection are:
  - Patient himself, the bacteria is present in the skin, nose, oral and perineum.
  - Cut down site.
  - Indwelling urinary catheter.
  - Hospital associated infection.
- Direct transfer is by
  - Droplets from coughing/sneezing.
  - Dust.
  - Water.
  - Hand -doctor/paramedical staff/relatives.
  - Mattress/sheets.
  - Dressing instruments/cheatle forceps.
- Blood stream -Intravenous line.
  - Host has three defenses-skin , leukocytes , and immune system
  - All the 3 mechanisms are impaired in burns.

Bacteria of the Burn Wound

- *Pseudomonas, Streptococcus, Staphylococcus, E. coli, Klebsiella.*

- The toxin liberated by these bacteria enter the circulation and affect the normal function leading to wound sepsis.
  - MRSA is common cause of infection in burn wound patients and usually spread by hands of staff members.
  - The MRSA can cause severe problem in immunocompromised patients.
  - Basic infection control procedures of hand washing, extensive cleaning and barrier nursing are not always sufficient to control infection.
  - A period of closure and disinfecting procedure has to be carried in addition.
  - Local wound MRSA efficiently eradicated by daily dressings with betadine/dakins.
  - Systemic life threatening infection treated with vancomycin or teicoplanin.
  - *Pseudomonas* is another hospital acquired resistant infection. Treated with betadine saline dressings.

20.4 LOCAL SIGNS OF BURN WOUND INFECTION (FIG. 20.1)

- Abscess formation.
- Black or brown local areas of discoloration.
- Conversion of second degree burns to third degree burns.
- Change of color-Purple, black, brown and blue.
- Discoloration is purplish round the margin of the wound.
- Erythema gangrenosa/eschar softening (Fig. 20.2)
- Enhanced sloughing/or early sloughing and rapid eschar separation of burned tissue.
- Focal signs of sepsis/foul smell/focal areas of discoloration.
- Green color of *Pseudomonas* infection/granulation deteriorating.
- Hemorrhagic patches in the subcutaneous tissue.

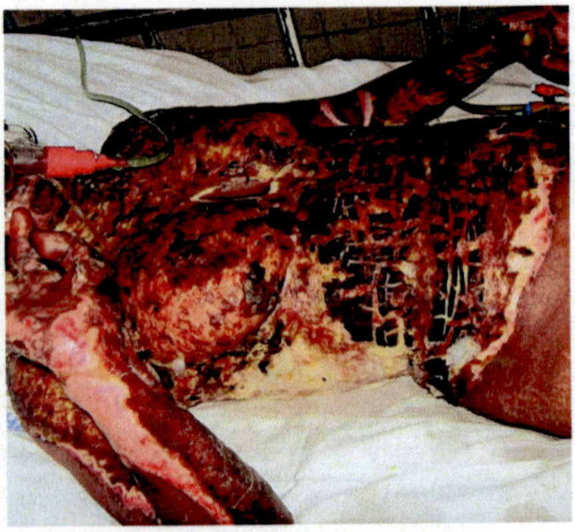

Fig. 20.1: Local signs of sepsis

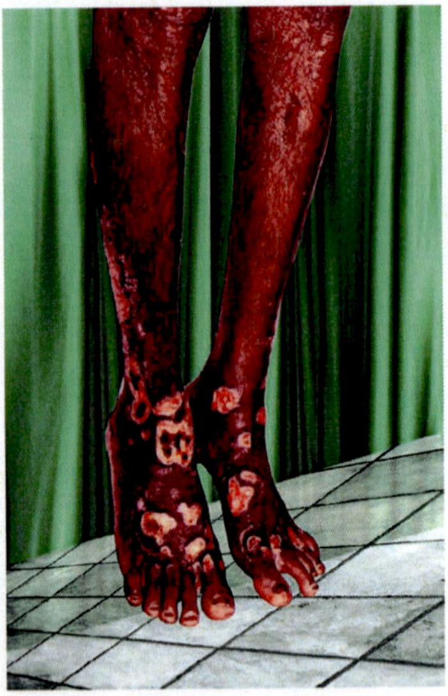

Fig. 20.2: Erythema gangrenosa

20.5 EFFECTS OF LOCAL WOUND SEPSIS

- Destruction of deeper tissue.
- Destruction of new epithelium.
- Destruction of skin graft.

20.6 POLICY TO FOLLOW (METHOD OF CONTROL OF BURN WOUND INFECTION)

- Improve general health by providing adequate nutrition.
- Good nursing care and techniques.
- Local wound care by early wound excision to remove all dead tissue and coverage.
- Immediate wound culture of burn wound for patients referred from other hospital.
- Isolation of patients, use of disposable material, regular hand washing with soap and water/betadine scrub followed by spirit washes.
- Regular and thorough cleaning of burn rooms and furniture with soap and water, lysol and dakins solution.

20.7 PREVENTION OF BURN WOUND COLONIZATION

Aseptic Measures

- Patients should have separate isolated rooms visitors restricted.
- Doctors and staff should wear a sterile cap mask gown and gloves before touching the patient.
- Before and after each procedure thorough hand washing with spirit or soap and water is stressed.
- Clean wounds should be dressed first.
- Avoid dropping the soiled dressing material on the floor.
- Keep separate bins for each room.
- Frequent cleaning and carbolization of rooms.

Local Treatment

- Daily cleaning the wound with saline and dressing with SSD (Silver sulpha diazene ointment).
- Removing the loose slough and if eschar is adherent to the deeper structures-grid escharotomy helps in separation (this method prevents blood loss).

Systemic Treatment

- Early recognition and aggressive therapy will help the burn patient to come out of sepsis.

The treatment priority follows the VIP format

V= Ventilation-Check respiratory rate get ABG (Arterial blood gas studies)
Start 40% venture -60% - CPAP
(Continuous positive airway pressure)

I = Infusion - Start IV fluids
- Give blood/plasma
- Amino acids
- Intralipids.

20.8 ROLE OF NURSE IN WOUND CARE

- Observe the color and odor of the dressing daily while doing the burn dressing.
- Report to the doctor immediately if there is any obvious change.
- Take the pus for culture and sensitivity, obtain the report.
- Change the topical antibiotic solution.
- Dressings should be changed twice or thrice a day to reduce the infection.

In Summary

- Wound sepsis remains feared sequelae in the patient who has suffered major burn injuries.
- The presence of large areas of devitalized ,necrotic tissue compiled with profound immune suppression sets the stage for rapid microbial proliferation in the wound and also into the normal adjacent tissues.
- This invasive burn wound sepsis unless treated energetically leads to septic shock with ensuring mortality.
- The most revolutionary approach to wound excision was developed by "Zora Janzekovic" from Yugoslavia.
- In 1968 she reported use of tangential excision in the early treatment of patients who had predominantly deep partial thickness burns of limited extent.
- This technique entails sequential removal of thin layers of the burned tissue until a viable graftable wound bed is developed or Shaving of successive layers of burn eschar until reaching viable tissue with pin point arterial bleeding.

- This technique allowed for improved intraoperative assessment of burn depth and for definitive wound closure at the same operative setting.
- The clinical benefit depends on immediate closure of the wound by either autografts, xenografts or any skin substitutes.

Chapter

21

SEPTIC SHOCK

21.1 INTRODUCTION

- Large open burn wounds containing necrotic tissue makes it susceptible to infection.
- The microorganisms multiply and colonize wounds easily due to the immunocompromised state of the patient.
- Infection and septicemia should be suspected when patient shows signs of disorientation, hyperpyrexia, hypotension, hypoxia, and tachypnea.
- Shock is defined as an abnormal physiologic state in which the flow of blood is insufficient to maintain adequate nutritive perfusion at the capillary level.
- Sepsis is defined as a spectrum of clinical conditions caused by the response of the patient to infection. It includes the full range of response from systemic inflammatory response to organ dysfunction to multiple organ failure and ultimately death.
- Septicemia is a state of microbial invasion causing signs of illness.
- The predominant feature of septic shock is arterial vasodilatation. An imbalance of homeostatic mechanism leads to DIC.
- There is a deficiency in several clotting factors due to consumption of these factors.
- Respiratory failure is the most important cause of death in patients with shock.

21.2 CLINICAL MANIFESTATION

Hyperventilation is the earliest sign. Disorientation, confusion, GI manifestation such as nausea, vomiting and diarrhea are other symptoms.

Chapter

22 ADULT RESPIRATORY DISTRESS SYNDROME

- A rising respiratory sign is the first to indicate that the patient is going into adult respiratory distress syndrome (ARDS).
- Lung injury is characterized by increased permeability of the alveolar membrane, diffuse alveolar damage, pulmonary edema, dyspnea, severe hypoxemia and pulmonary infiltrates.

Blood Gases

Although most cases of respiratory failure can be recognized by careful clinical examination, arterial blood gas studies gives an accurate measure of the severity of respiratory failure and of the response to treatment. Also shows reduced oxygen and normal CO_2.

Investigations

Chest X-ray appears clear at first and later hazy due to interstitial edema. Patchy infiltrates may also be seen.

22.1 NURSING ASSESSMENT

Early recognition of ARDS includes:

- History of burn injury in a closed space.
- Presence of facial burns.
- Soot in the mouth, pharynx and nose.
- Singed nasal hairs.
- Altered consciousness.
- Rising respiratory rate.

22.2 SIGNS AND SYMPTOMS

Respiratory Problems

- Cough
- Tachypnea
- Hoarsness
- Strider
- Dyspnea
- Wheezing
- Decreased lung compliance.

Cardiac Problems

- Tachycardia, arythmias, angina.

Neurologic

- Fatigue
- Vertigo
- Ataxia
- Headache
- Confusion
- Hallucinations.

22.3 DIAGNOSTIC STUDIES

- Arterial blood gas studies
- Carboxy hemoglobin level
- Fiberoptic bronchoscopy
- Chest X-ray
- Electrolyte
- Pulmonary artery and wedge pressure
- Pulse oxymeter.

22.4 MEDICAL MANAGEMENT

- Prophylactic intubations
- Continuous positive airway pressure
- Humidified oxygen
- Physiotherapy

- Mechanical ventilation
- Careful circulatory support
- Nutritional support.

22.5 PHARMACOLOGICAL TREATMENT

- Infusion- Start IV fluids to maintain perfusion.
- Transfuse blood, plasma, amino acids, intralipids to prevent circulatory collapse.
- Pulmonary specific vasodilators like dopamine are started in small doses to maintain renal perfusion.
- Appropriate antibiotics used based on bacteriological monitoring of the burn wound.
- Topical antibiotic used generously twice a day for local wound care.

22.6 SPECIFIC NURSING MANAGEMENT

- Promoting adequate ventilation
- Providing safety interventions
- Encouraging rest
- Monitoring vital signs
- Reducing anxiety
- Delivering nursing care in a calm and reassuring manner
- Administering drugs promptly
- Document patients responses

Treatment of ARDS

- With better understanding and management of sepsis importance is given to early recognition and immediate aggressive therapy to reduce progression to full blown septicemia.
- Treatment priority follows the VIP format that is—ventilation, infusion and perfusion.
- A rising respiratory is the first indication of sepsis.
- An arterial blood gas study done at this stage indicates a low partial pressure of oxygen.

- **Ventilation:** Considering that ventilation has the highest priority importance is given to administering oxygen to keep the arterial partial pressure at about 80-100 mm of Hg.
- **Infusion:** In septic shock circulating volume can decrease significantly as fluid shifts into the interstitial space and hence rapid infusion of electrolyte solution, colloid, amino acids, fatty acids and 10% dextrose should be given to prevent circulatory collapse.
- **Perfusion:** Adequate oxygen and fluid replacement helps in maintaining or improving perfusion. In addition vasodilating drugs like dopamine are started in small doses to maintain renal perfusion.
- Appropriate antibiotics are started based on bacteriological monitoring of the burn wound.
- Topical antibiotic is used generously twice a day for local wound care.
- In addition close monitoring of respiratory rate, pulse rate, blood pressure and urine output is maintained.
- Patient who do not respond to this simple increase of fractional inspired oxygen concentration and continue to have refractory hypoxemia are to be treated with continous positive airway pressure (CPAP) this mode of treatment obviates the need for endotracheal intubation and the subsequent infection.
- **CPAP:** This is an effective supportive therapy in hypoxic respiratory failure. It increases oxygenation without intubation. Patient is able to communicate.
- A number of measures are necessary in the treatment of sepsis in burn patients, such as correct local care, nutritional support , environmental control and surgical therapy. All are necessary for effective treatment.

22.7 INHALATION INJURY

Burn injuries are often associated with inhalation injury which greatly increases their risks for post burn pneumonia and mortality. Patients who have a history of injury in a closed space or facial burns are more likely to have inhalation injury.

- The pathophysiology of inhalation injury is complex. It is classified into three types based on anatomic location.
- The first type includes upper-airway injuries caused primarily by thermal injury to the mouth, oropharynx and larynx.
- The second type includes lower airway and parenchymal injuries (e.g. tracheal, bronchial, and alveolar injuries) caused by chemical and particulate constituents of smoke.
- The third type includes metabolic asphyxiation, which is the process by which certain smoke constituents impair oxygen delivery to or consumption by the tissues.

Physical Examination

Findings-burns of the face, carbonaceous sputum, soot in the nose and mouth, wheeze, rales, rhonchi, voice change, corneal burn, signed nasal vibrissae , cough, strider, dyspnea, intraoral burn.

22.8 CONCLUSION

Success in ARDS Management is Achieved by

- Accurate early recognition of ARDS.
- Quick initiation of treatment.
- Careful monitoring.
- Specific problem based care.
- Prompt medication.
- Periodic evaluation.

22.9 ROLE OF NURSE IN PATIENTS WITH ARDS

Identify the first clinical sign of ARDS -tachypnea . The respiratory rate will gradually increase from the base line reading and this is the most important sign to say that the patient is going in for an impending ARDS . Identifing this sign and informing the treating surgeon is a very important task of the burn nurse.

At this time treating the patient as if the patient has gone into full blown septicemia is important. Early recognition and aggressive treatment is the only chance to bring the patient out of sepsis.

Saturation should be maintained (connect to pulse oximeter). ABG (arterial blood gas) studies should be done and if saturation is less connect to 40% venture, another ABG is sent after two hours of 40% venture, most often saturation returns to normal, so continue with the same management.

Start IV fluids. Maintain intake/output chart and vital signs every 15 minutes, administer antibiotics as per order, and maintain hourly urine output.

Chapter 23

OXYGEN THERAPY

Anyone who is hypoxic requires oxygen therapy. Several techniques are available to administer oxygen including masks, nasal prongs or naso pharyngeal catheters.

23.1 MASKS

- Fixed performance masks.
- Variable performance masks.

Fixed Performance Masks

- Also called venturi masks.
- They deliver an accurate fixed concentration of oxygen at a high flow rate.
- Models are available to deliver-24%, 28%, 35%, 40%, or 60% oxygen.
- Such masks are useful when we need to provide an exact percentage of oxygen.

Variable Performance Masks

These include all other masks and provide a flow of oxygen which the patient breathes along with air drawn in from around the outside of the mask.

23.2 NASAL PRONGS

These deliver oxygen at the nostrils and depends on the oxygen being carried down through the nose during inspection. They are inefficient if the patient is breathing through the mouth.

23.3 NASAL PHARYNGEAL CANNULA

This is a piece of soft tubing which is inserted into the nasopharynx. The cannula is inserted into the nose until the tip appears below the soft palate and then taped at the nose. This method can cause gastric distention . The safest way to use these cannulae is with a T piece which allows any excess pressure to be blown off.

In patients who are ventilated the addition of PEEP (positive end expiratory pressure) is used when ever more than 50% oxygen is required.

23.4 HUMIDIFICATION

Oxygen is dry and may cause an uncomfortable drying of the mucous membrane therefore water humidifier is used to over come this problem.

Nebulizers

These devices produce very small droplets of liquid drugs when a flow of oxygen is passed through them. When the patient breathes the oxygen, the drug passes to the bronchi where it either acts directly or is absorbed . The most common drugs used in this way are the bronchodilator drugs such as salbutamol, and terbutaline.

Chapter 24

FACE MASK CONTINOUS POSITIVE AIRWAY PRESSURE

Most of the severe burn patients go into sepsis associated with hypoxemia which does not respond to a simple increase in oxygen concentration by using venture masks . Earlier these patients were all intubated and ventilated with a high risk of infection.

We describe our method of treating such patients with continous positive airway pressure (CPAP) with out any infective complications.

Discussion

CPAP is a breathing system which supplies a continuous flow of gas to generate a constant airway pressure while the patient is spontaneously breathing. Patients who do not respond to a simple increase in oxygen therapy require intubation and ventilation which eventually causes damage to the lungs.

With CPAP mask therapy endotracheal intubation and ventilation is avoided. It provides an effective means of improving oxygenation in refractory hypoxemia. Lung complications are reduced because it is invasive.

CPAP therapy is traditionally administered by endotracheal tube using ventilators.

CPAP mask circuits helps burn patients who have sepsis with refractory hypoxemia.

These patients are alert and have good ventiltory effort proved by low $PaCO_2$ values while breathing spontaneously. Thus one can avoid endotracheal intubation and ventilation which has a high infection rate. Mask therapy is suitable in these patients because of its invasiveness and chances of acquiring respiratory infection are thus reduced.

24.1 DESIGN OF CPAP

Figure 24.1 depicts the design of CPAP

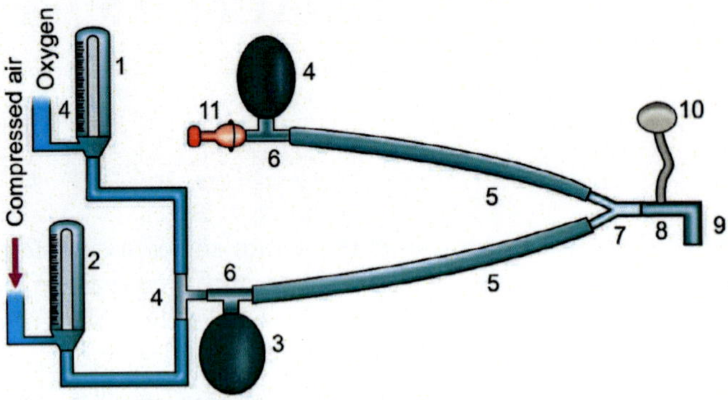

		Quantity
1.	Oxygen flow meter	1
2.	Air flow meter	1
3.	3 liter reservoir bag	1
4.	2 liter reservoir bag	1
5.	Corrugated tube 80 cm x 2.2 cm	2
6.	T-piece	3
7.	Y- connector	1
8.	Connector with side tube	1
9.	Swivel mount	1
10.	Pressure manometer	1
11.	Expiratory pressure valve	1

Fig. 24.1: Design of CPAP

Chapter

25 HYPERTROPHIC SCAR AND KELOID

25.1 SCAR

- The word scar is derived from the Greek word eschara.
- Scar is a fibrous tissue and replaces normal skin after destruction of dermis.
- Scar occurs when deep thick layer of skin is damaged. Deeper the damage worser the scar.

25.2 KELOID

- The word keloid is derived from the Greek word "chele or crab's claw."
- It is characterized by lateral growth into the normal skin. It is raised, itchy, and painful.
- Skin damage due to trauma, surgery, acne can cause keloid formation.

25.3 CLINICAL FINDING

- Elevated due to extracellular matrix
- Itching due to histamine production by mast cells
- Redness due to increased vascularity.

25.4 CLINICAL DIFFERENCE

HYPERTROPHIC SCAR (Figs 25.1 to 25.3)	KELOID (Figs 25.5 and 25.6)
• Increased inflammatory phase of healing	Remains elevated
• Confined to original site	Extends onto the normal skin
• Regress spontaneously	Recurrence is common
• No recurrence	
• Treatment is by using silicone gel pressure and excision	Treatment is by steroid injections excision followed by radiotherapy

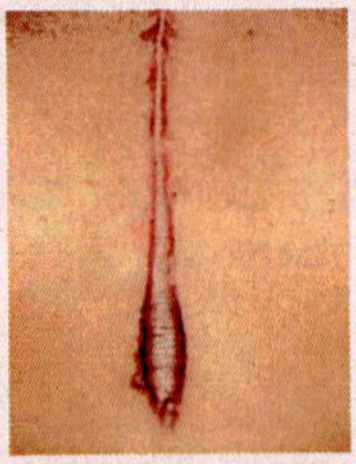

Fig. 25.1: Suture line hypertrophic scar

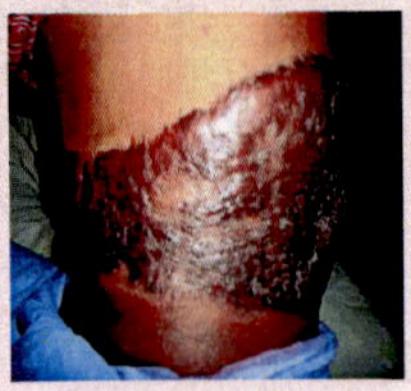

Fig. 25.2: Hypertrophic scar over

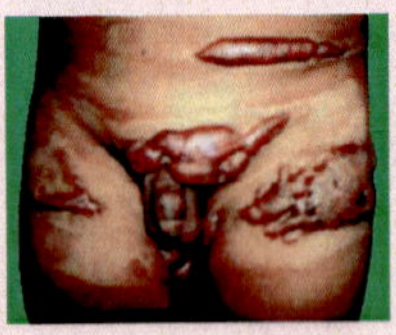

Fig. 25.3: Hypertrophic scar over burn site

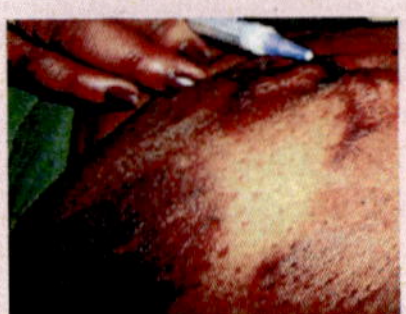

Fig. 25.4: Injection kanacort for hypertrophic scar

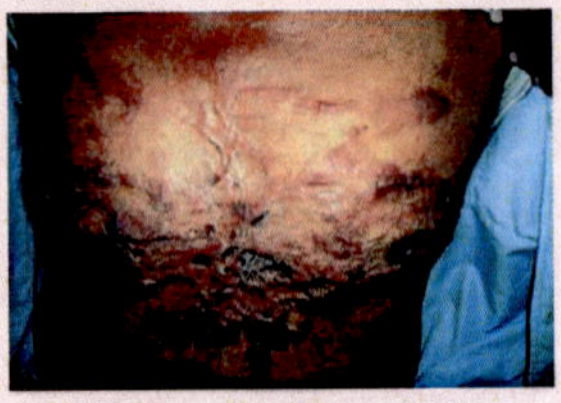

Fig. 25.5: Keloid chest

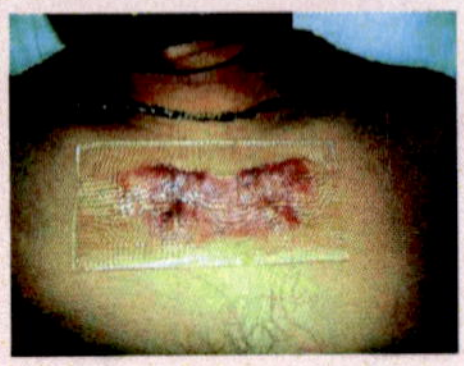

Fig. 25.6: Silicone gel sheet donor site over keloid scar

25.5 PROBLEMS ASSOCIATED WITH ABNORMAL SCARS

- Cosmetic problem.
- Contracture.
- Loss of function over joints.
- Painful and itchy.

25.6 TREATMENT

Pressure Therapy

Compression Treatment Includes

- Elastocrepe bandage
- Pressure garments
- Button compression
- Pressure ear rings.

Procedure

- Use as early as possible
- Applied for 24 hours
- 10-15 minutes release for cleaning
- Continue for 6-12 months.

Advantages

- Reduces edema
- Reduces cohesiveness of collagen
- Accelerates scar maturation.

Disadvantages

- Compliance is poor
- Blister under pressure garments
- Minimal effect on old scar.

Silicone Gel Sheet

- To be used 24hrs a day
- Washed and reapplied
- Scar becomes soft, flattened and pain free.

Action

Hydration, occlusion, rise in temperature causes change in adhesion molecules.

Disadvantage

Contact dermatitis, pruritus, rashes and maceration.

Contratubex Ointment

- Antiproliferative
- Anti-inflammatory
- Softening and smoothing action
- Effective in case of indurated hypertrophic painful scar.

Intralesional Steroid Injections

- Reduced collagen synthesis
- Reduced production of inflammatory mediators and fibroblasts
- Dose -10-40 mg/ml, intralesional
- 20G needle
- Response 50-100%,
- Recurrence 9-50%

Contraindication

- Skin infection

Adverse Effects

- Depigmentation
- Atrophy
- Necrosis
- Cushing syndrome.

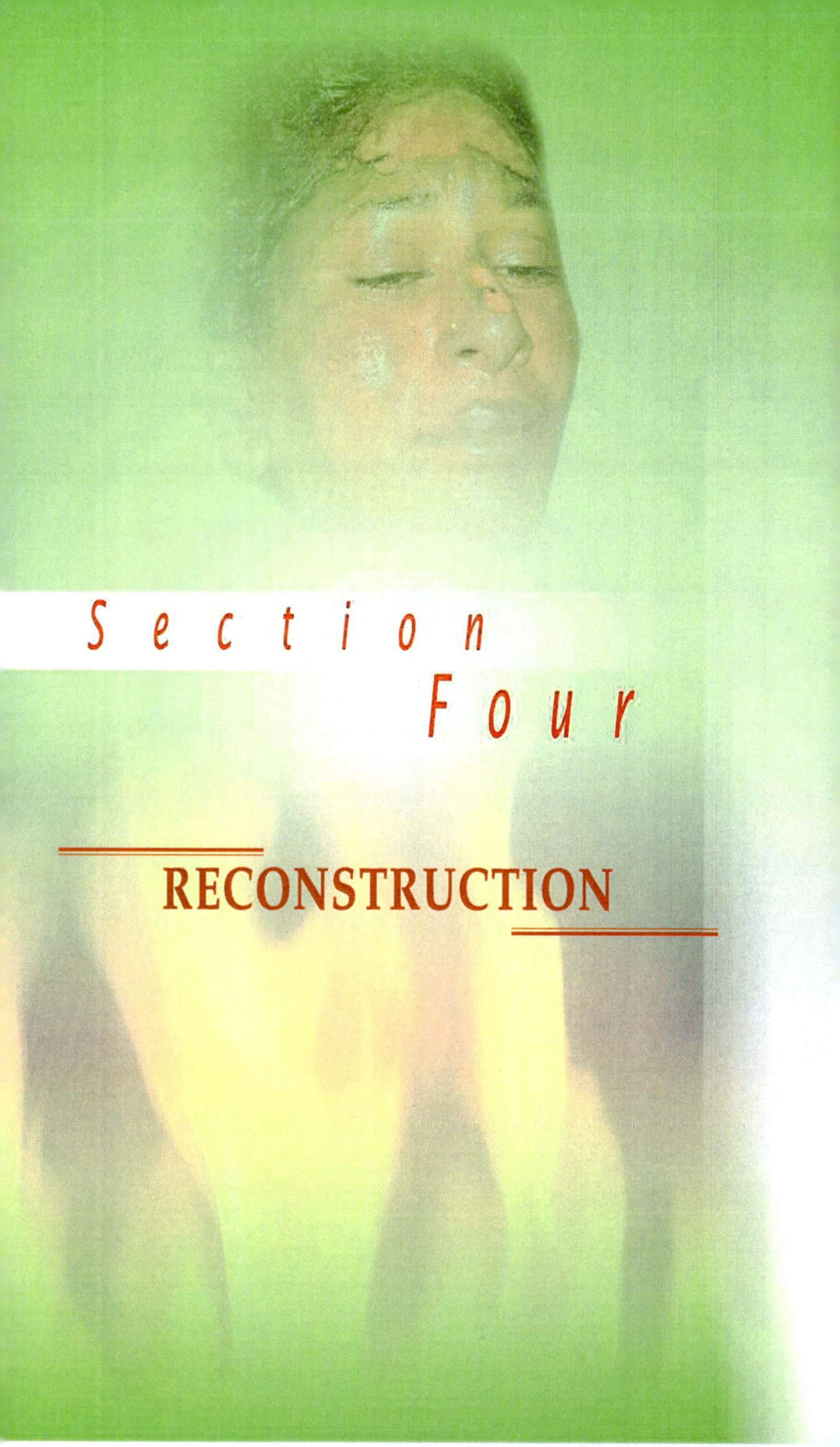

Section Four

RECONSTRUCTION

Chapter

26 RECONSTRUCTIVE PHASE

Reconstruction of a burn patient is a complex and a lengthy process that usually starts at the time of initial injury and often lasts from years to a lifetime. The useful techniques during the acute phase which help to minimize late reconstructive problems include:

- Active and passive mobilization and ambulation as soon as possible.
- Elevate and splint all limbs and joints.
- Start rehabilitation and pressure therapy as soon as possible.

Non Surgical Approach to Burn Reconstruction

- Compression by elastic bandage, tubular bandage and custom fitted garments.
- Silicone gel.
- Steroids.
- Masks and splints.

In spite of all this, contractures and scarring remain.

Surgical Treatment

Surgical treatment can be classified into essential surgery and desirable procedures:

Essential Surgery

It is performed to preserve important functions. Exposed cornea requiring eyelid reconstruction (ectropion correction). Contracture of the neck that causes problem for general anesthesia. Oral contracture that interfere with anesthesia, hygiene and eating.

Desirable Procedures

It includes the type of reconstruction a patient wants. At this time patient's priorities are the most important. Example nose, burn alopecia and scar revisions. These are performed after scar maturation has occurred.

Conclusion

Burn reconstruction is a very rewarding field. For most problems there is either a simple solution or a complex solution. As burn team workers, we can all help the burn survivors to face the society with confidence.

Chapter

27 BURN CONTRACTURE

Burn contracture is a very difficult problem as it results in severe functional deformity.

27.1 TYPES OF CONTRACTURES

Intrinsic contracture (Figs 27.1 and 27.2)

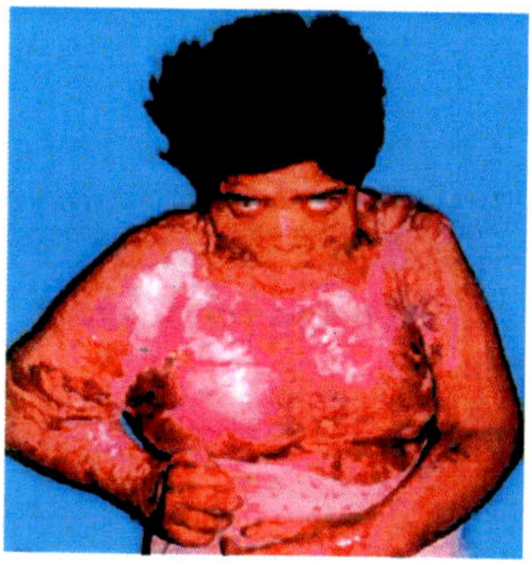

Fig. 27.1: Intrinsic contracture of neck and lip

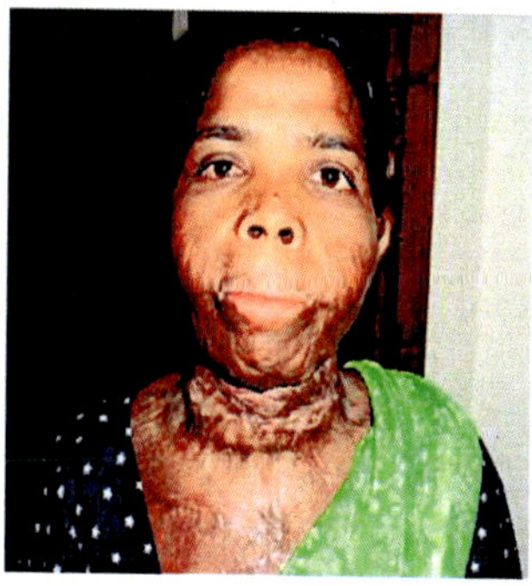

Fig. 27.2: Release of neck and lip contracture

Extrinsic contracture (Figs 27.3 to 27.5)

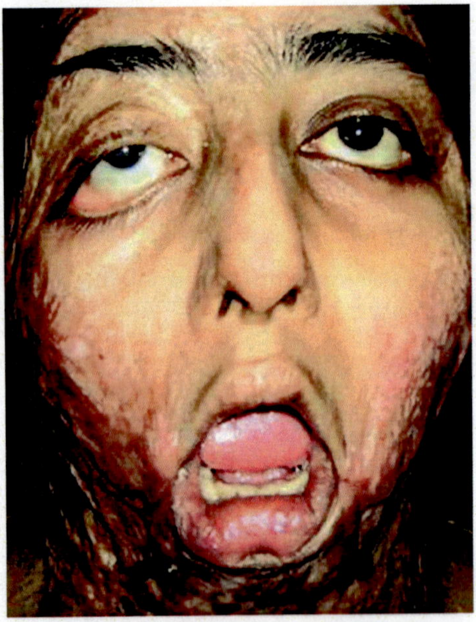

Fig. 27.3: Extrinsic contracture of eyelids

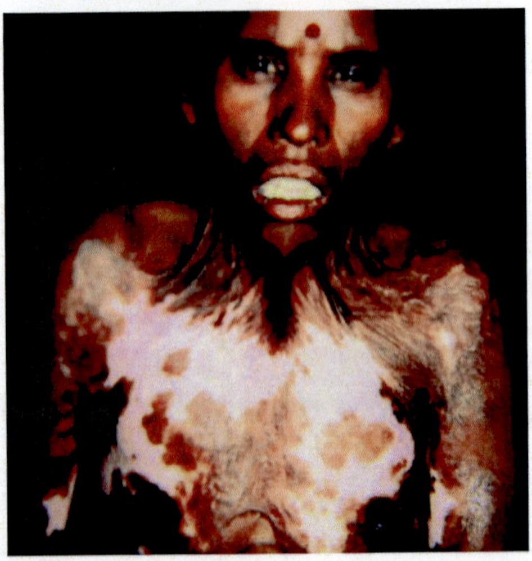

Fig. 27.4: Extrinsic contracture of lower lip

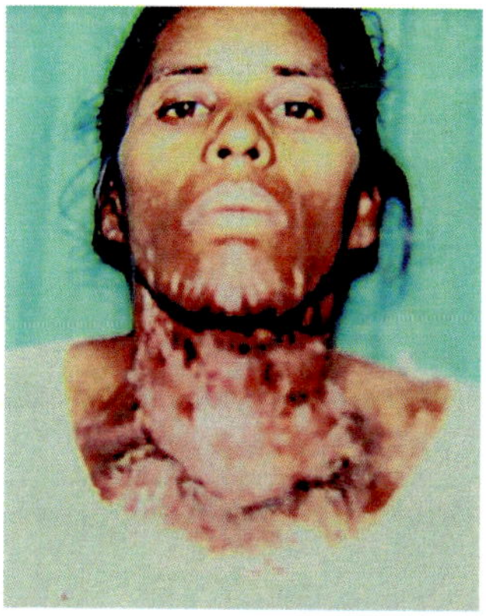

Fig. 27.5: Correction of lower lip after neck release

Intrinsic Contracture

When the contracture is in the deformed structure and responsible for the deformity then it is called intrinsic contracture. For example, neck and lip contracture distorting the neck and lip only.

Extrinsic Contracture

When the contracture band is away from the deformed structure and is indirectly responsible for the deformity by traction or pull over the normal skin then it is called extrinsic contracture. For example, when there is a contracture of the neck and lip, but the eyes get pulled down due to the traction of the normal skin on the cheek.

Chapter

28 BURN RECONSTRUCTION

1. Burn reconstruction is very complex and challenging in a developing country like India , because of the many hurdles like poor compliance, no regular follow up, hot climate, non availability of splints and garments and financial constraints.
2. The strategies to over come these hurdles are:
   - Firstly to use local flaps when ever and where ever possible.
   - Secondly simple innovative inexpensive and easily available devices and splints should be used.
   - Thirdly use simple techniques which does not require compliance or follow up. For example,
   - Suction tube as nostril retainer for nostril stenosis (Figs 28.1 and 28.2).
   - Tea strainer as a protective ear cup (Fig. 28.3).
   - Wooden spatulas as mouth spreader after microstomia correction (Fig. 28.4).
   - Sponge roll as collar (Fig. 28.5)
   - Emery paper as dermabrader (Fig. 28.6)
   - Elastocrepe bandage with Velcro as chin strap for pressure (Fig. 28.7)

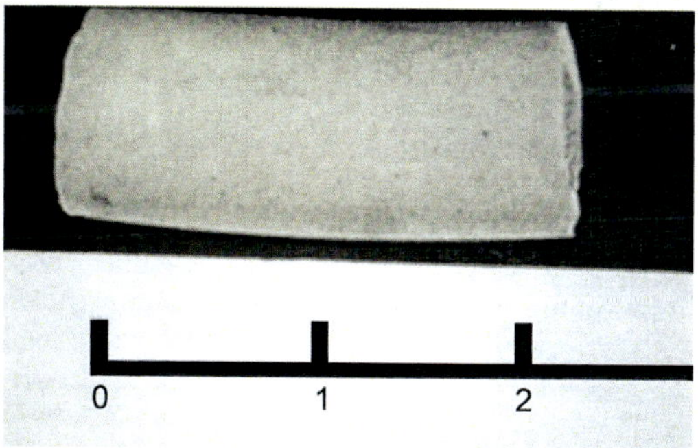

Fig. 28.1: Rubber tube

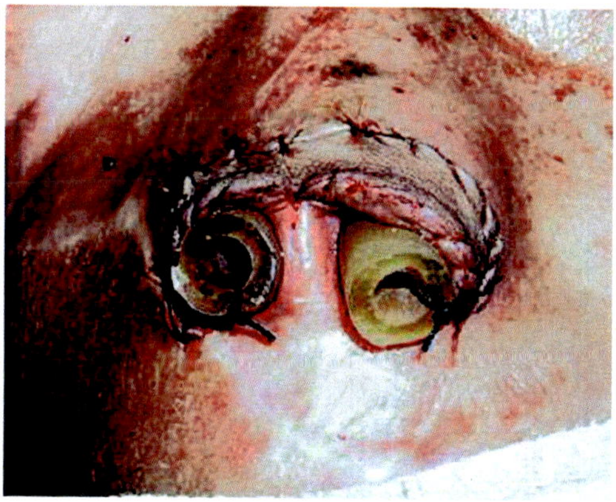

Fig. 28.2: Rubber tube as nostril retainer

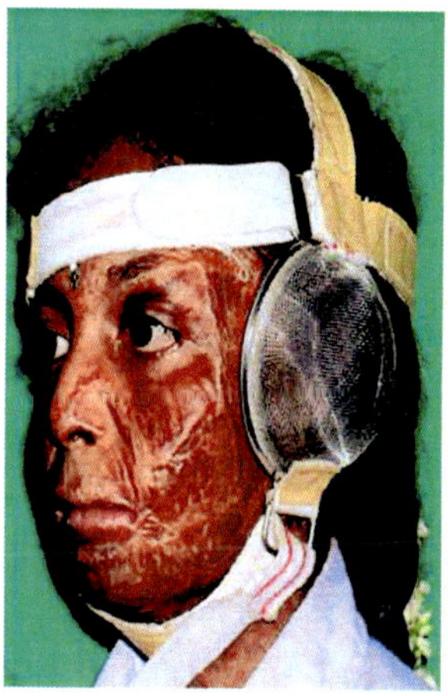

Fig. 28.3: Tea strainer as ear cup

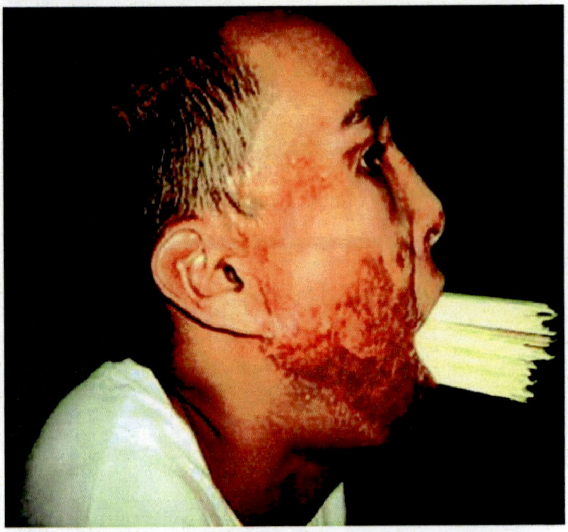

Fig. 28.4: Wooden spatula as mouth spreader

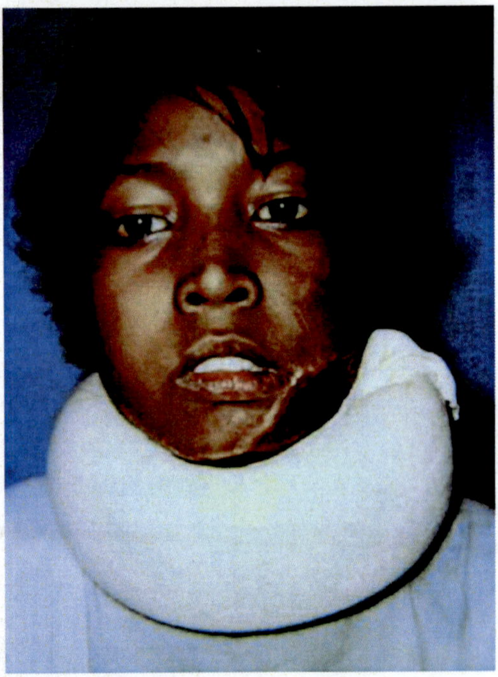

Fig. 28.5: Sponge roll as collar

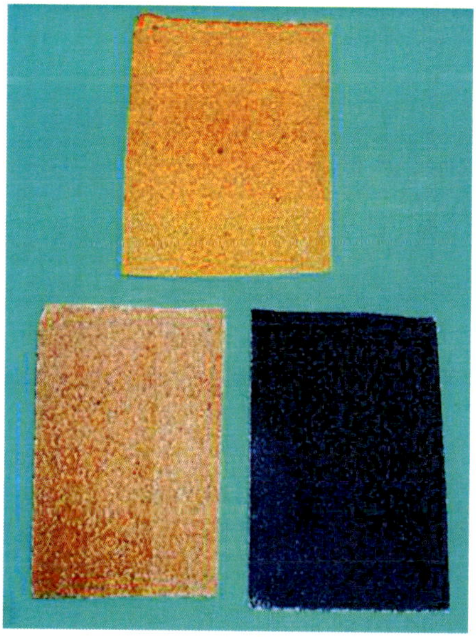

Fig. 28.6: Emery paper as dermabrader

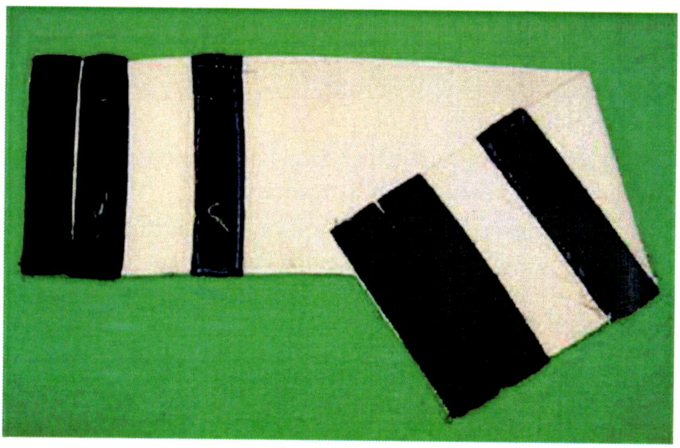

Fig. 28.7: Elastocrepe bandage with velcro as pressure garment

Burn reconstruction is a very rewarding field. The surgical challenge of reconstruction takes on an importance almost unmatched in any other area of reconstruction. We can help our patients to face the society with confidence.

Chapter 29

RECONSTRUCTIVE PRINCIPLES DURING ACUTE PHASE

- Reconstruction of a burn patient is a complex and a lengthy process that usually starts at the time of initial injury and often lasts from years to a lifetime.
- Excellent patient surgeon relationship is very essential to gain confidence and cooperation of the patient, and for this the initial surgery performed should demonstrate improved results and also if need be multiple simultaneous procedures should be done.
- Though priority is prevention of deformity followed by reconstruction of active and passive function. It is the involvement of the reconstructive surgeon in the acute care of the injury which is of paramount importance.
- The useful techniques during the acute phase which help to minimize late reconstructive problems.
- Start active and passive mobilization and ambulation as soon as possible.
- Elevate and splint all limbs and joints.
- Use darts to prevent linear contracture across joints.
- Place grafts seams that follow skin lines.
- Place grafts on joints transversely.
- Use sheet grafts whenever possible.
- Avoid widely expanded mesh grafts.
- Excise and graft all wounds that do not heal in 3 weeks of injury.
- Use cosmetic units when necessary.
- Start rehabilitation and pressure therapy as soon as possible.
- Nonsurgical approach to burn reconstruction includes compression by elastic bandage, tubular bandage and custom fitted

garments. Silicone gel, steroids, masks and splints. In spite of all this contractures and scarring remain leading to conflict in the timing of surgical reconstruction.

- The psychology and rehabilitation prefer early reconstruction where as the wound biology favors late reconstruction. Even though it is more rewarding to do reconstructive procedures on the mature scar, in the patient's best interest, it is best not to wait for scar maturation.

29.1 RECONSTRUCTIVE PRINCIPLES AREA WISE

Face

This is a controversial subject. The reconstructive surgeon must be involved in the acute care of burn injury to prevent functional deformity. Excision and grafting of facial burns that have not healed in 15 days time are taken up for grafting. The graft seams are placed along skin lines, custom made face masks are worn continuously to give pressure evenly (Fig. 29.1).

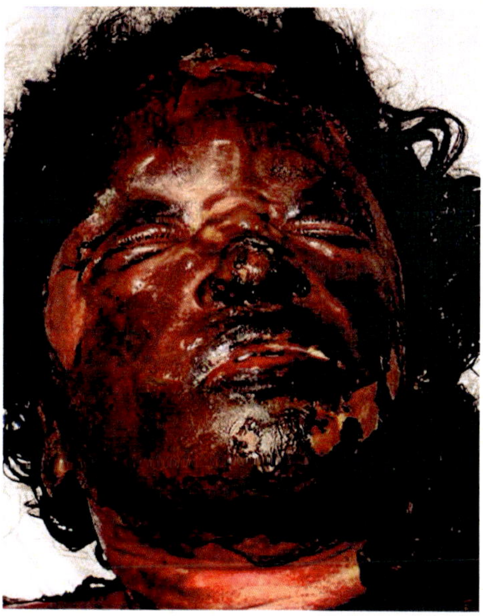

Fig. 29.1: Acute facial burns

Eyelid Reconstruction

This can be extrinsic or intrinsic. A very important consideration is to eliminate extrinsic causes of ectropion before concentrating on the eyelids. It is possible for contracture of the face and neck to transmit forces to the eyelid causing secondary problems. Once extrinsic problems are corrected the residual ectropion should be corrected, one at a time either upper or lower as over correction is imporotant. It is preferred to use full thickness skin grafts for lower eyelid and thin for upper eyelid (Figs. 29.2 to 29.6).

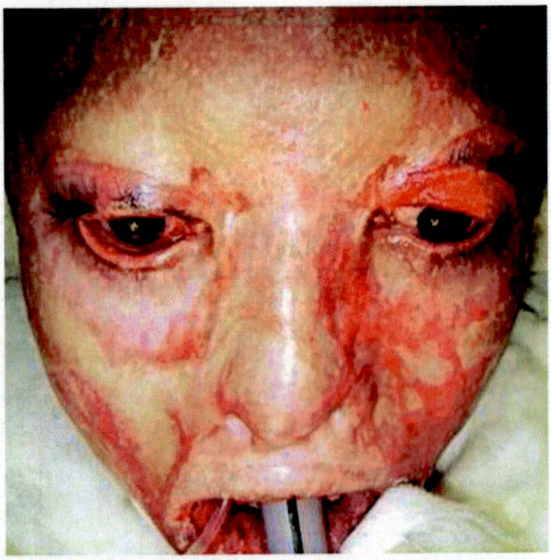

Fig. 29.2: Upper eyelid ectropion

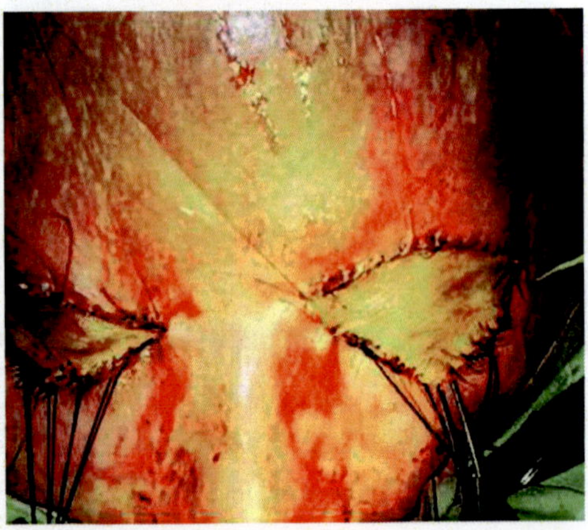

Fig. 29.3: Upper eyelid correction with skin graft

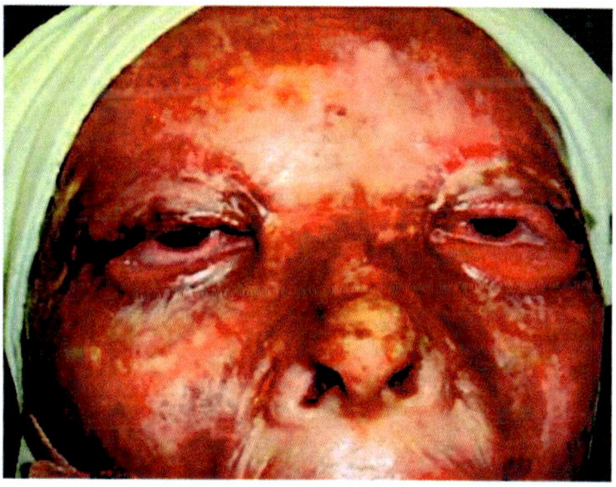

Fig. 29.4: Lower eyelid ectropion

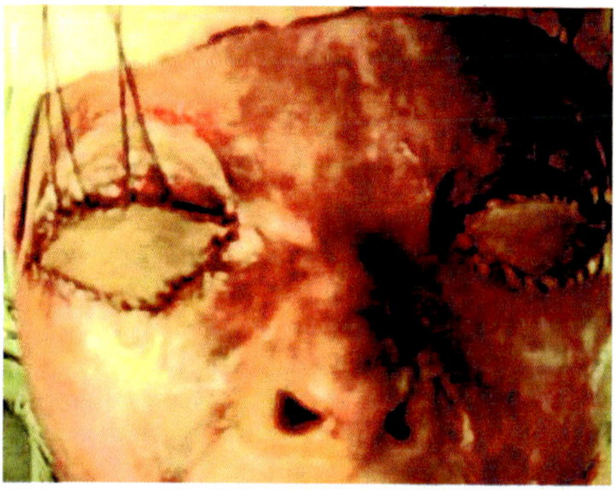

Fig. 29.5: Lower eyelid correction with graft

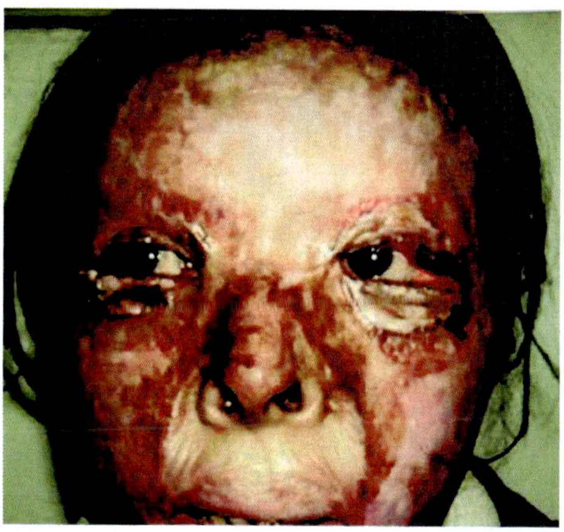

Fig. 29.6: Final result on 10th post op day

Ear Reconstruction

Although scarred tissue complicates ear reconstruction, there are several advantages of burn ear over a congenital ear. The burn deformity of the ear has all of the cartilage but folded by contraction. Simple release of which is sufficient to give a natural appearance. The total absence of the helical rim is reconstructed with rib cartilage graft and temporalis flap. The advent of vascularized temporal fascial flap has been a major boon for burn patients. Ear lobe are often adherent to adjacent neck skin. Simple division and closure is all that is needed for correction (Figs 29.7 to 29.10).

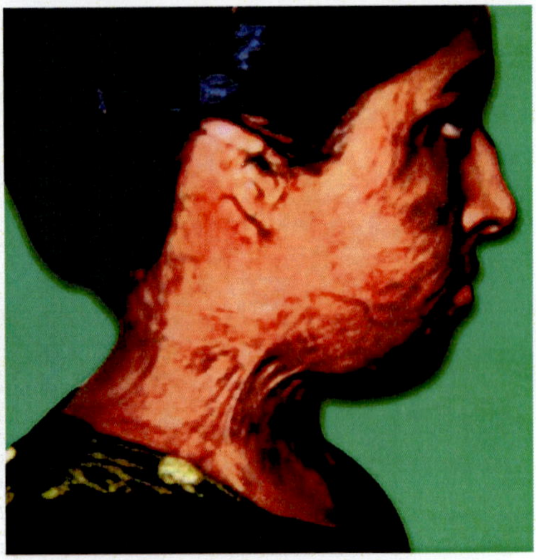

Fig. 29.7: Ear deformity

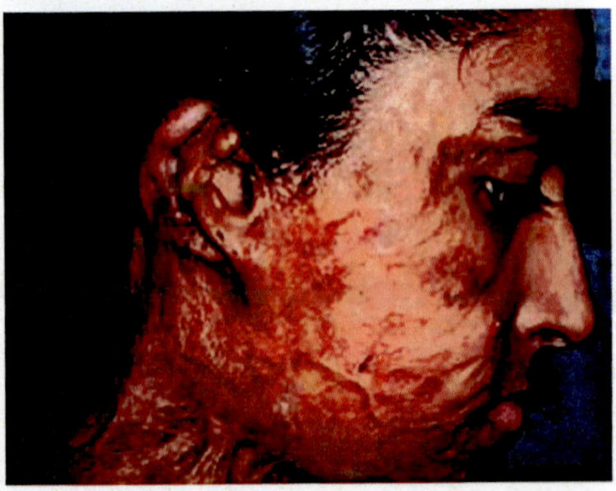

Fig. 29.8: Reconstruction with rib cartilage

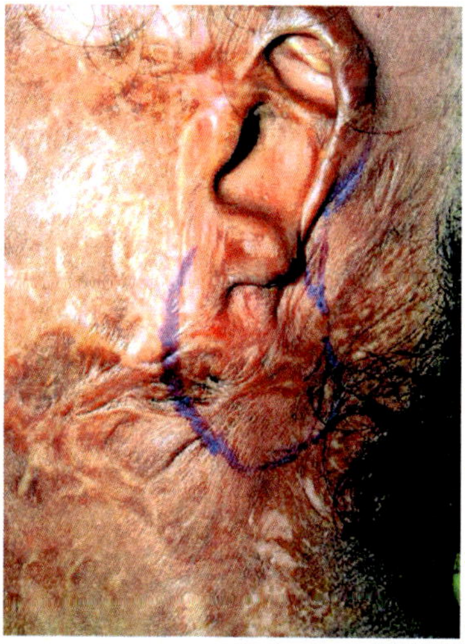

Fig. 29.9: Loss of ear lobe

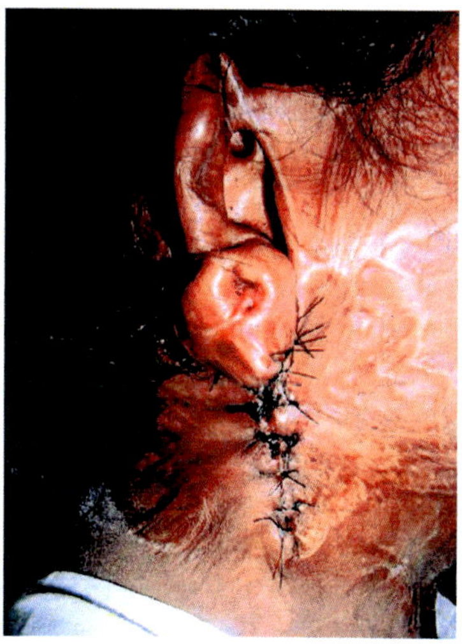

Fig. 29.10: Reconstruction of ear lobe from scarred burned tissue

Nasal Reconstruction

The greatest projection and central point of the face is the nose and successful correction is crucial to the patient's self image. Two common deformities of the nose are Nasal ectropion corrected with turn down flaps and full thickness skin grafts (Figs 29.11 to 29.14).

Nasal Stenosis

The scar removed and skin graft is sutured around a splint and placed in position for 6 months. Suction catheters have been found to be a very useful alternative for splints (Figs 29.15 to 29.17).

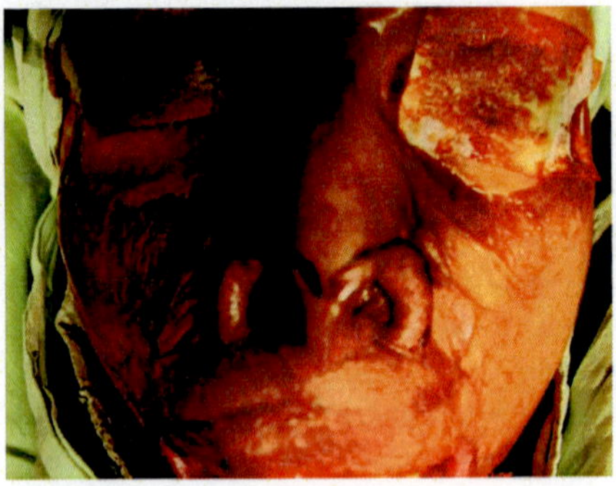

Fig. 29.11: Typical burned nose ectropion

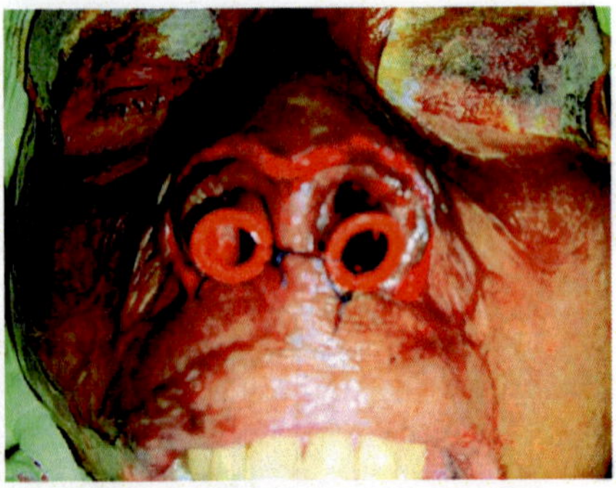

Fig. 29.12: Release ectropion and insertion of tubes

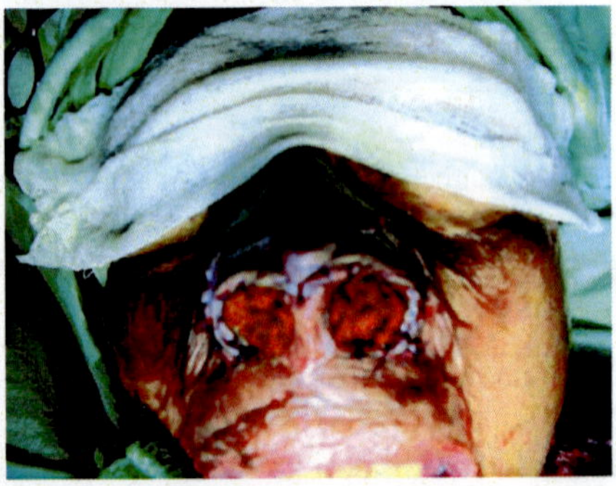

Fig. 29.13: Post op picture with graft in place

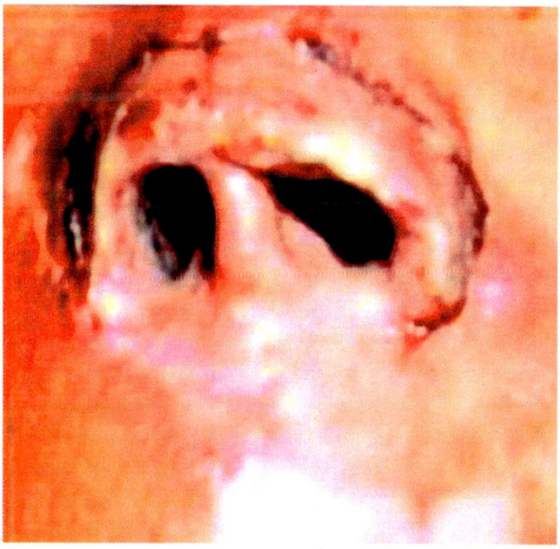

Fig. 29.14: Post op correction nasal ectropion

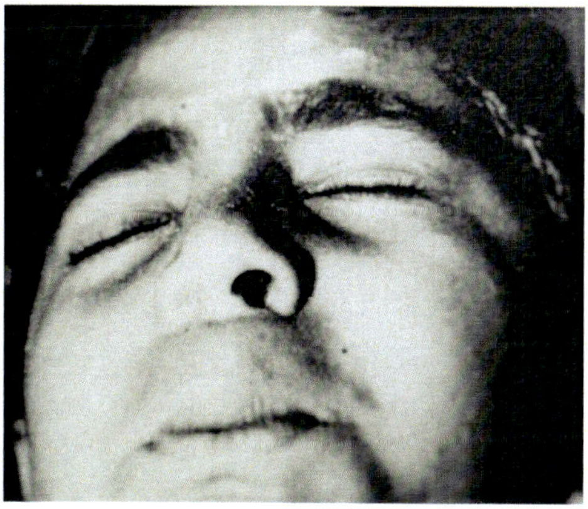

Fig. 29.15: Nostril stenosis

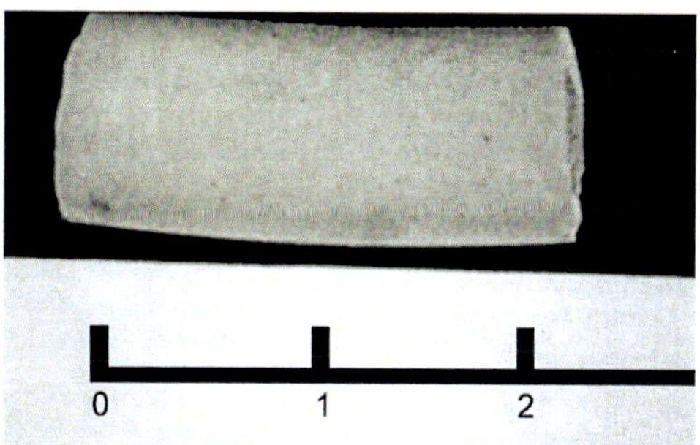

Fig. 29.16: Rubber tube as splint for 6 months

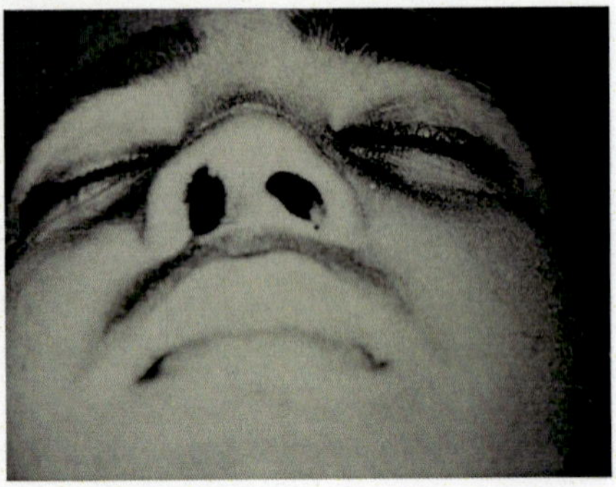

Fig. 29.17: Release stenosis and graft

Oral Commissure

Lateral margin of oral commissure which is at the end of nasolabial fold is determined. A triangular section of scar tissue is removed and the vermilion flap is transposed. Splints are crucial (Figs 29.18 to 29.20).

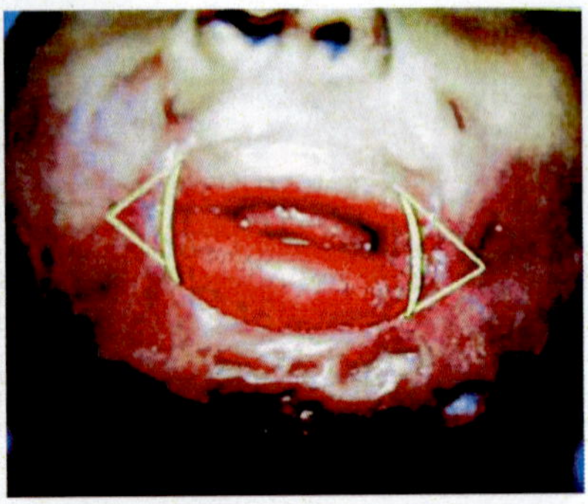

Fig. 29.18: Bilateral tight commissures

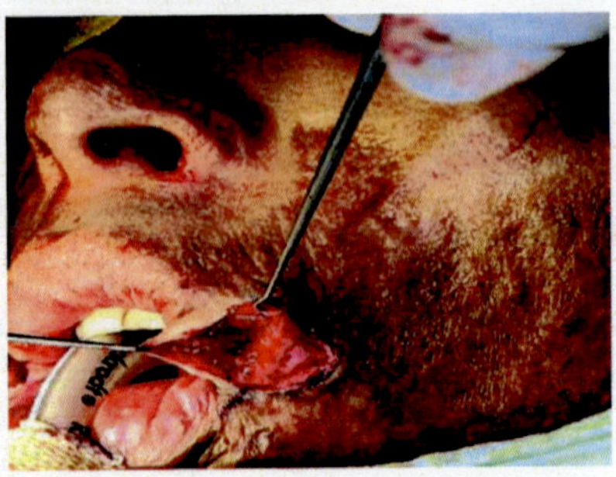

Fig. 29.19: Releasing the tight orbicularis muscle

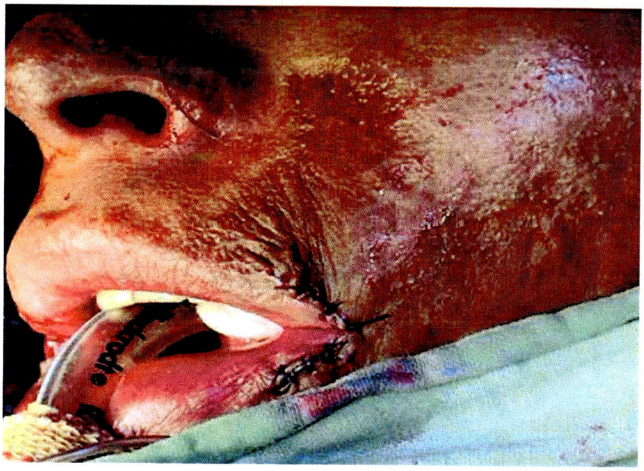

Fig. 29.20: Reconstruction of angle of mouth

Lower Lip

Ectropion is corrected by release of the lower lip. Partial vermilion-ectomy and wedge excision of the excess vermilion to maintain tension of muscle. The raw surface is covered with FTSG (Figs 29.21 to 29.23).

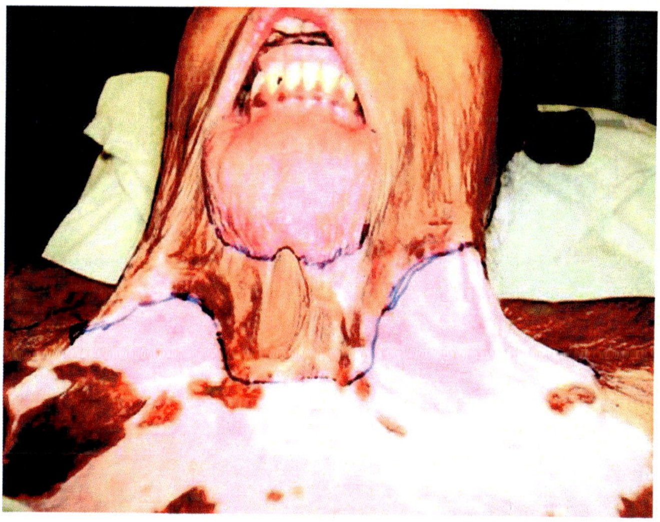

Fig. 29.21: Severe lower lip ectropion

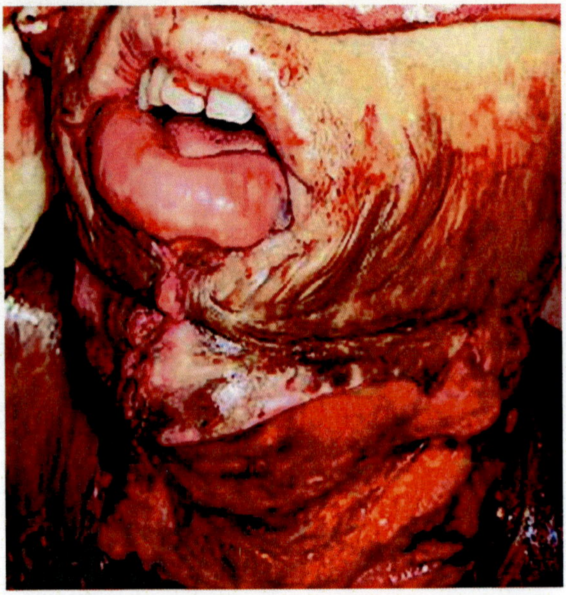

Fig. 29.22: Correction of lip

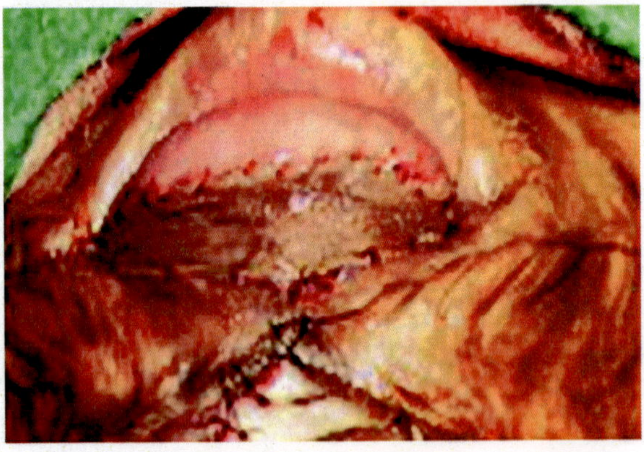

Fig. 29.23: Final result

Neck Contracture

Despite its obvious limitation, skin grafts are most commonly used in extensive neck contractures. A nasogastric tube for feeding and immobilization by post OP splinting is very essential for a good take (Figs 29.24 to 29.28).

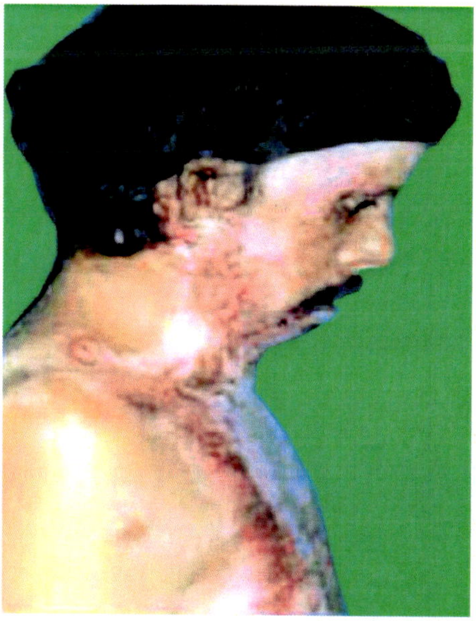

Fig. 29.24: Neck contracture

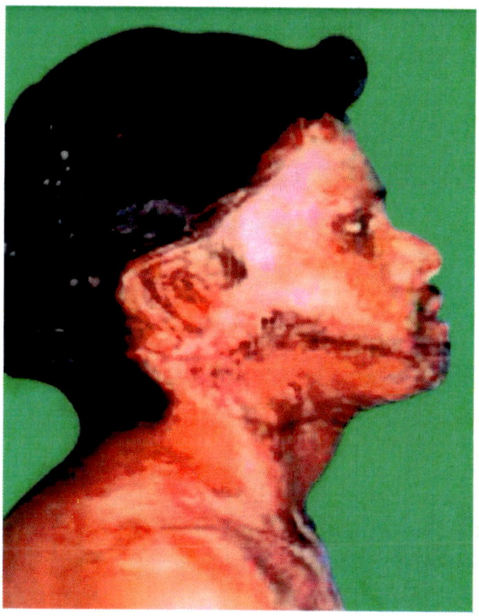

Fig. 29.25: Post release neck contracture with graft

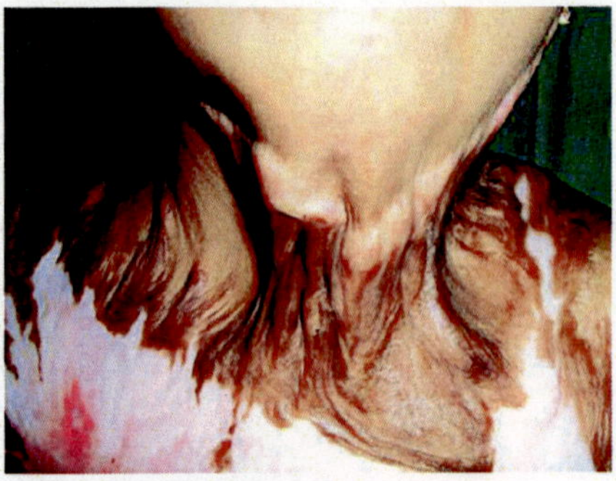

Fig. 29.26: Neck contracture

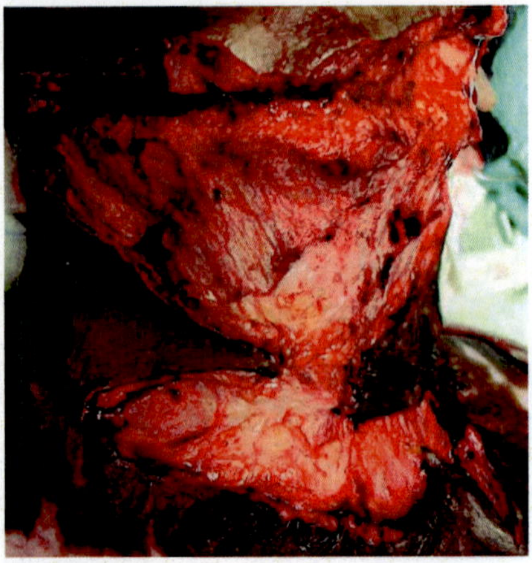

Fig. 29.27: Release contracture

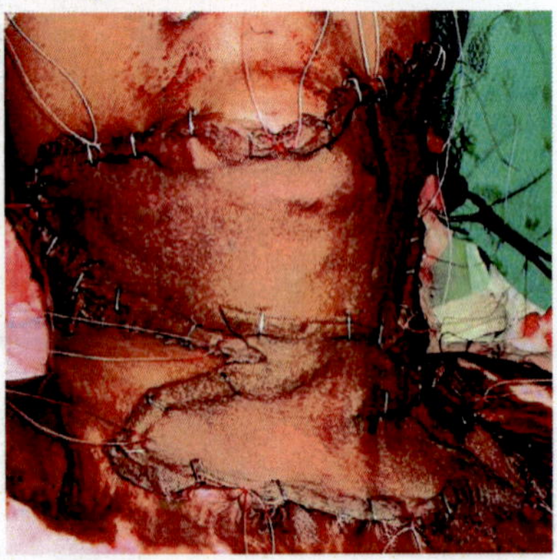

Fig. 29.28: Skin graft on raw area

Axilla

The scar band can be either anterior or posterior which can be corrected by release burn scar contracture and reconstruction with local flaps rather than using skin grafts, as unburnt tissue is always available in the axial itself. If need be parascapular fascial flap can be a useful alternative (Figs 29.29 to 29.32).

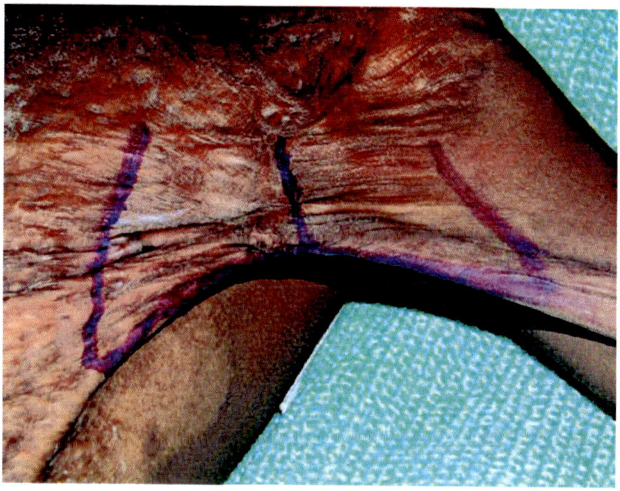

Fig. 29.29: Contracture of axilla

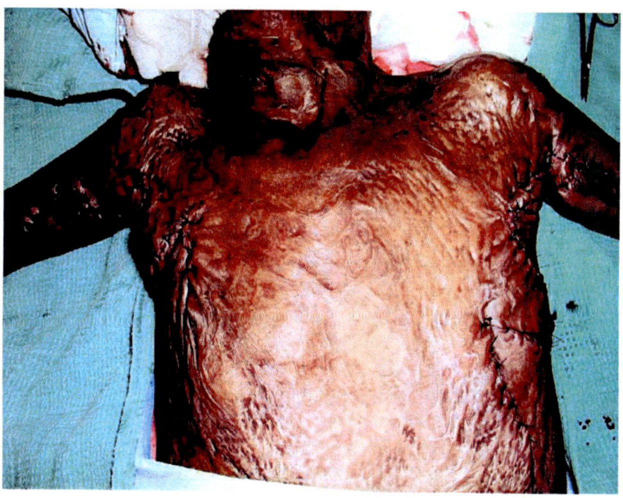

Fig. 29.30: Group1 release with 5 flap plasty

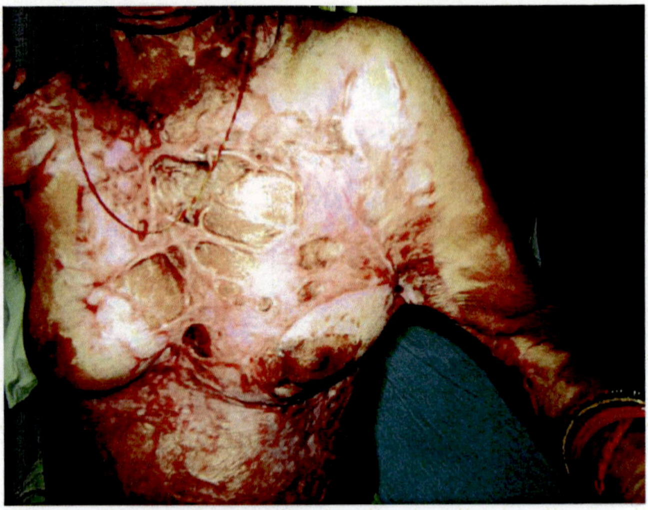

Fig. 29.31: Axilla contracture

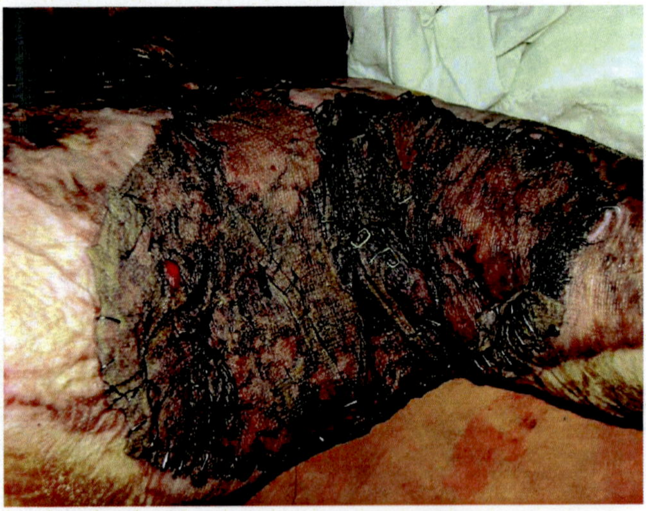

Fig. 29.32: Graft after release

Lower Extremity

It creates a unique problem splinting with early skin grafting prevents most of these contractures. However if contraction does occur, it is released using vertical and transverse incisions, k-wire fixation and resurfaced with STSG (Figs 29.33 to 29.39).

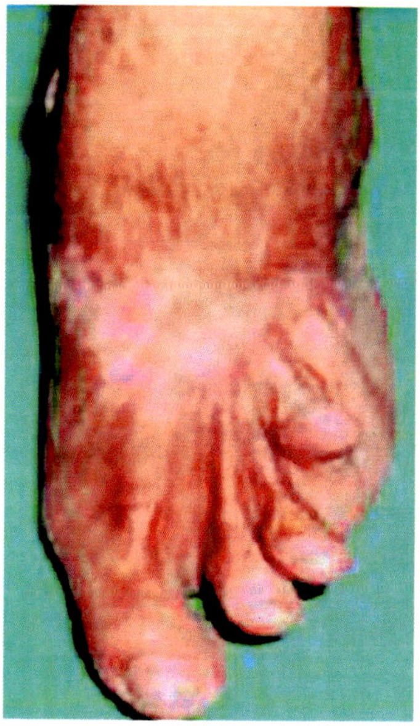

Fig. 29.33: Post burn scar contracture foot

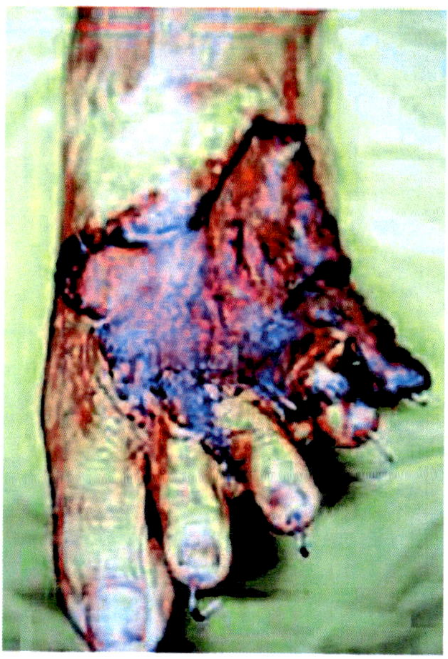

Fig. 29.34: Release contracture and graft

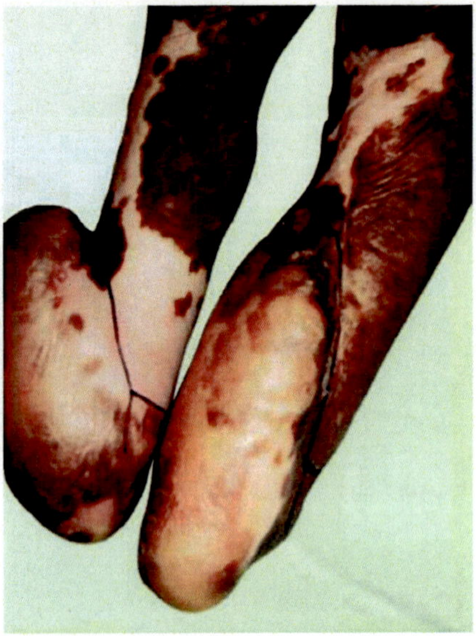

Fig. 29.35: Lower leg contracture

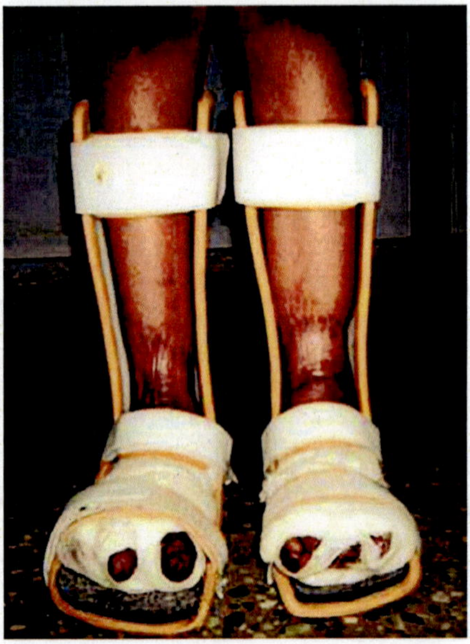

Fig. 29.36: Lower limb after correction

Breast

The goal is esthetic recontouring of the breast secondary procedures like nipple and areolar reconstruction is done at the peripubertal age. Surgical release of the breast is carried out by inverted T incision and resurfaced with split thickness skin graft. Silicone inserts and sternal straps help to improve scarring and shape (Figs 29.37 to 29.39).

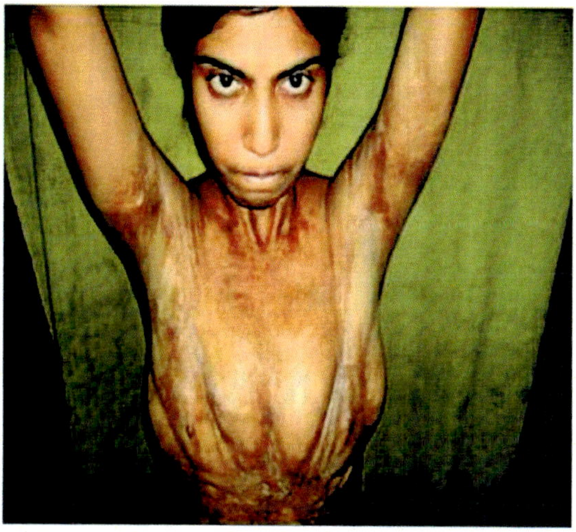

Fig. 29.37: Breast entrapped due to scar

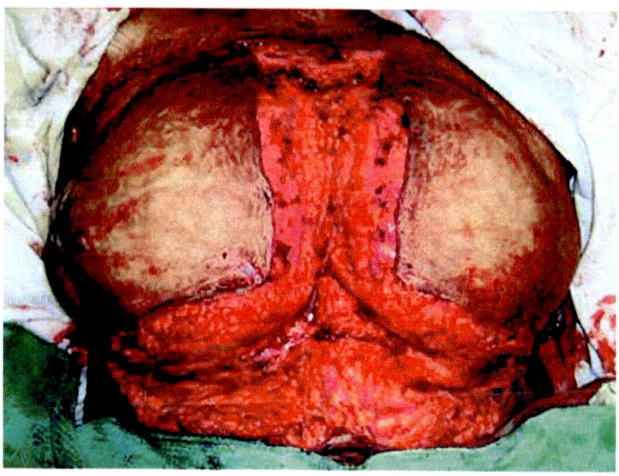

Fig. 29.38: Breast release

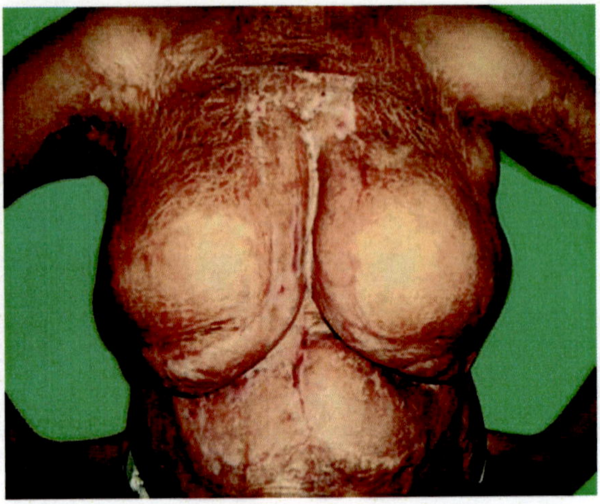

Fig. 29.39: Final result

Perineal Contractures

They are very common and can be corrected by local flaps (Fig. 29.40).

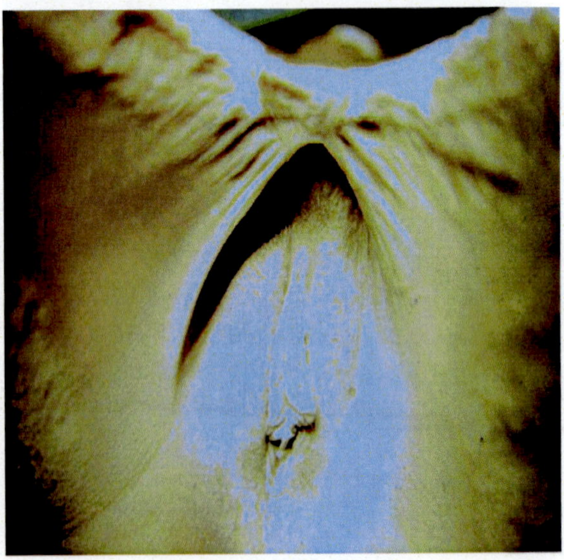

Fig. 29.40: Perineal contracture

Chapter 30 POST BURN AXILLARY CONTRACTURES

30.1 INTRODUCTION

Shoulder has the greatest range of motion of any joint. Maintaining that posses many problems for the burn team. Early splinting, positioning and motion of the arm to prevent contractures are very important.

Post burn axillary contractures should be corrected as soon as the diagnosis is established in order to avoid deeper tissue involvement. Several techniques have been defined to release the post burn contracture of the axilla. Axillary region is important because it has multi-directional activity. Scar contractures restrict various movements. Patients have problems with daily activities.

Scar tissue usually extends to the chest, back and upper arm compounding the restrictions.

30.2 CLASSIFICATION

Axillary contractures are classified into 3 groups depending on the involvement of the axillary fold.

Group I

Involving only the anterior or posterior axillary fold (Figs 30.1 to 30.8).

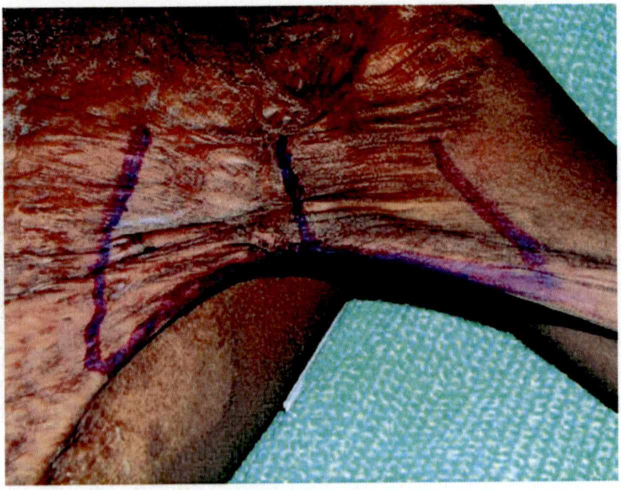

Fig. 30.1: Group1 axillary contracture

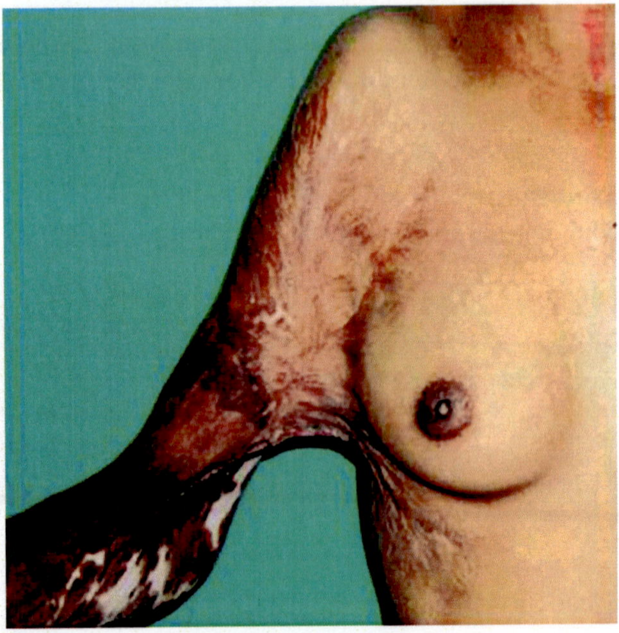

Fig. 30.2: Anterior fold only

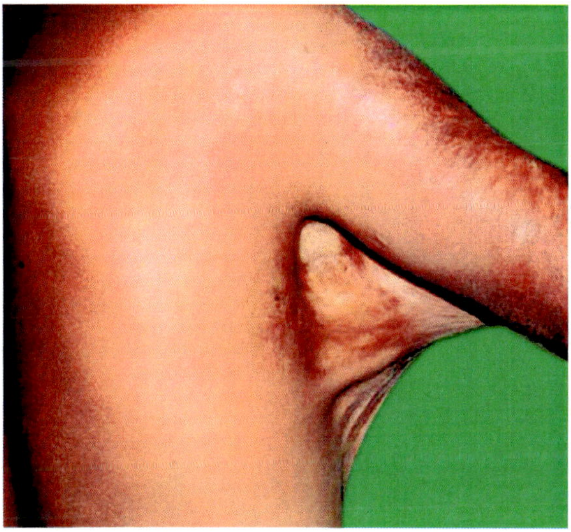

Fig. 30.3: Showing only anterior fold involvment

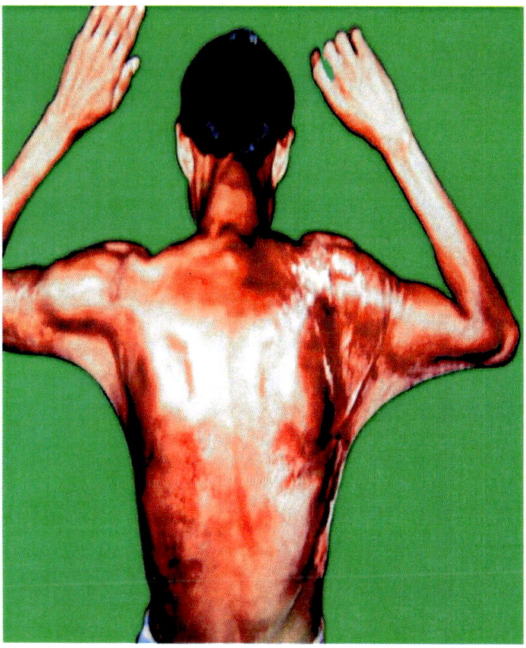

Fig. 30.4: Anterior and posterior fold involved

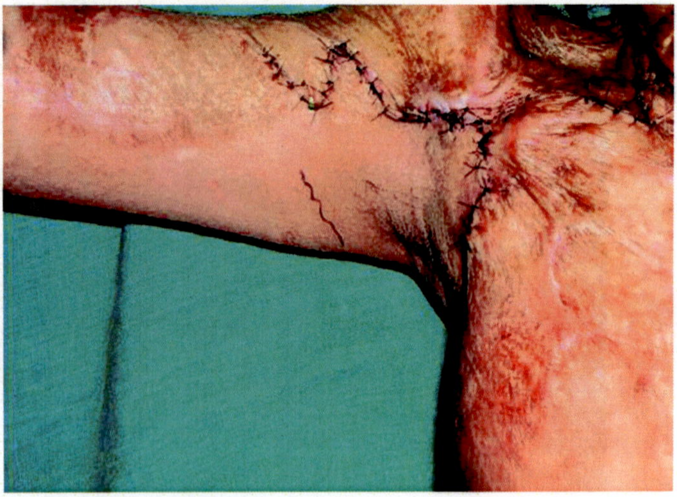

Fig. 30.5: After four flap correction

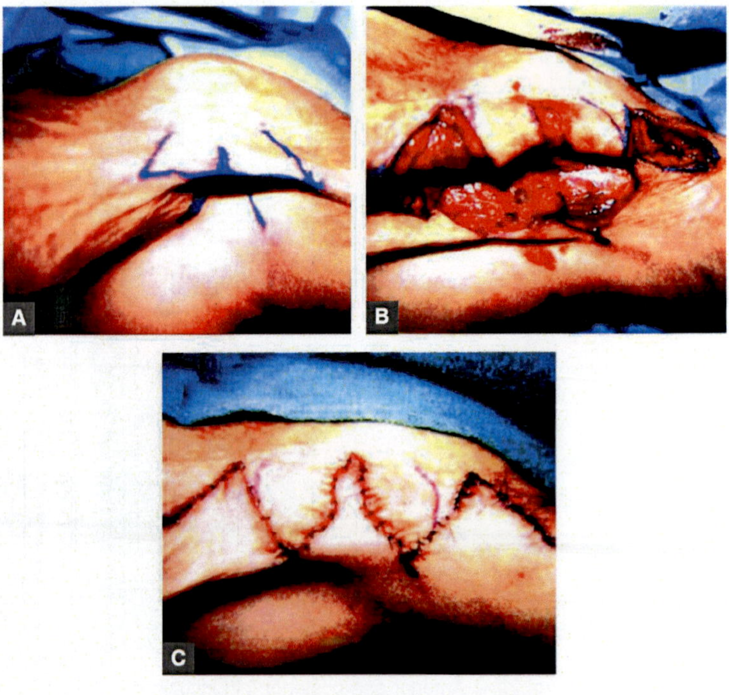

Figs 30.6 A to C: Five flap correction

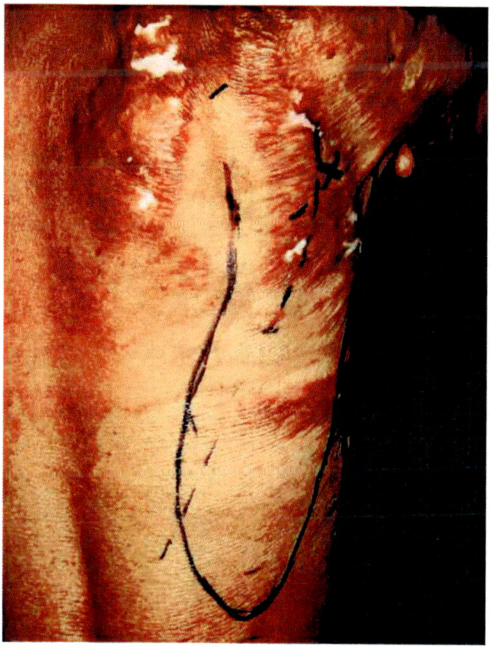

Fig. 30.7: Teated by parascapular flap

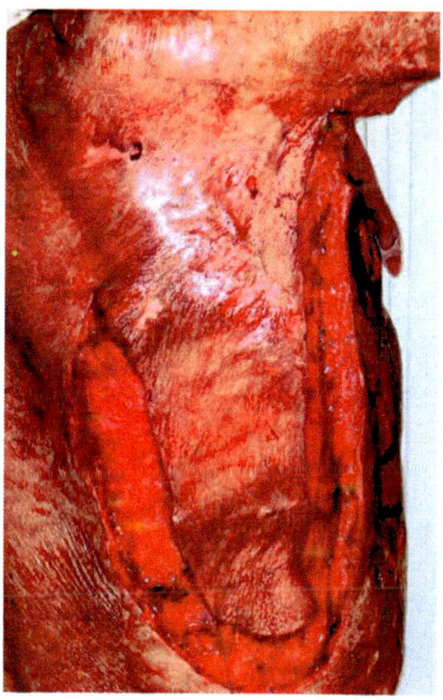

Fig. 30.8: Parascapular flap raised

Group II

Involving both the anterior and posterior fold but sparing the apex of the axilla (Fig. 30.9)

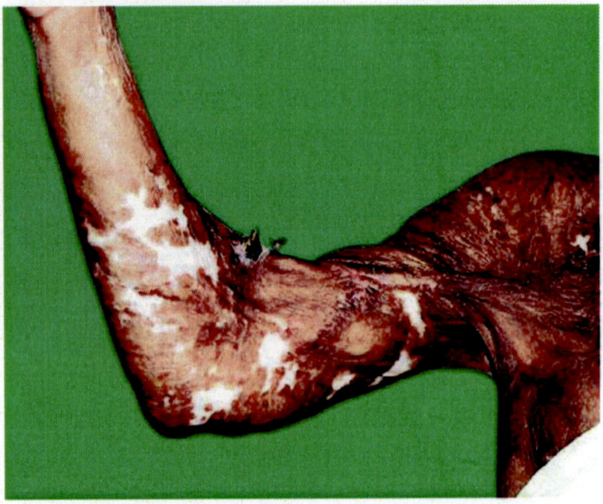

Fig. 30.9: Group II- Both folds involved

Group III

Most severe deformity where the complete axilla is involved and attached to the chest wall (Figs 30.10 to 3.12).

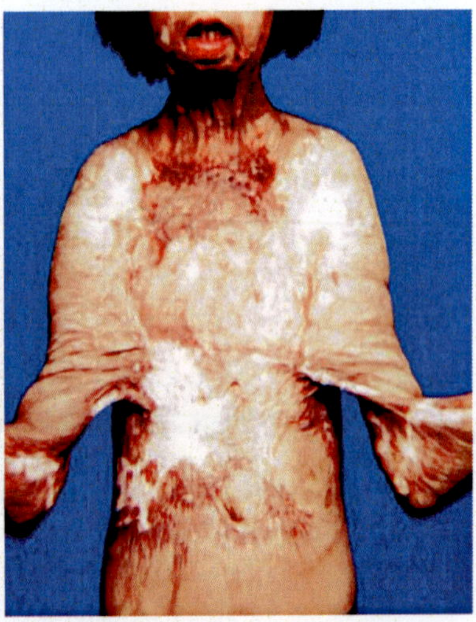

Fig. 3.10: Group III-Severe contracture involving both folds and chest

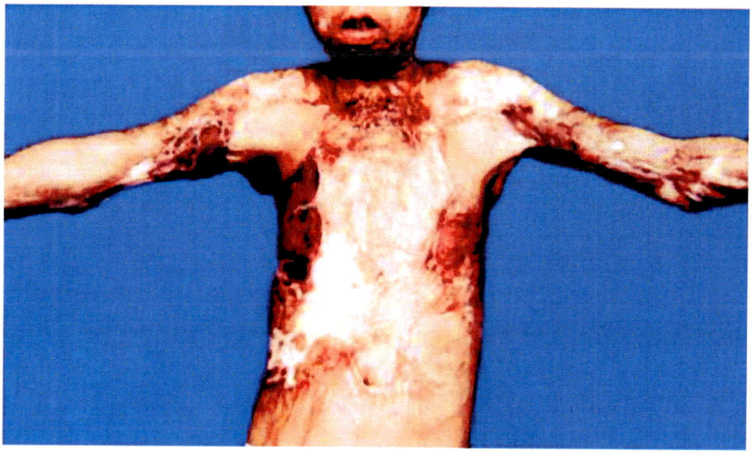

Fig. 30.11: Release bilateral contracture

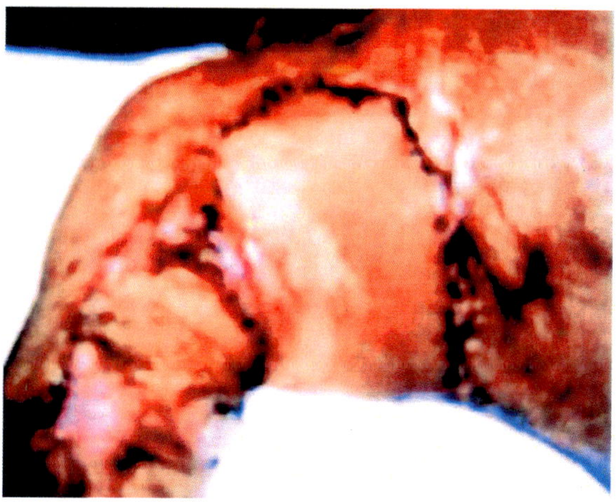

Fig. 30.12: Parascapular flap

30.3 TREATMENT

a. Simple local flaps
b. Transposition flaps
c. Regional faciocutaneous flaps
d. STSG.

The only condition which requires grafting is, when there is extensive raw area either on the chest or arm on release.

Considering that skin grafts for post burn contracture release of the axilla has a high recurrent rate, flaps have been the best choice. Generally normal skin is mandatory to raise flaps, we perform flaps which are reliable, safe and simple even when skin is burnt. The use of flaps have been an invaluable option in preventing re-contractures.

We know that reconstruction of scar contracture is a challenge for plastic surgeons. We use subcutaneous pedicle flaps for correction of scar contractures and early release to avoid deeper tissue involvement. Including subcutaneous tissue as a pedicle in the flap has increased the survival of flaps.

Scar bands of either anterior or posterior axillary fold are corrected by utilizing unburnt skin to break up the scar band using multiple Z plasties. The major short coming of Z plasty is that scarring at the base will jeopardize the circulation and tip necrosis is often found. This can be avoided by using deeper dissection subcutanoues pedicle flaps.

For severe contractures a regional flap like latissimus dorsi flap should be considered.

30.4. ADVANTAGES

- Postoperative immobilization is shortened.
- Postop therapy is reduced.
- Hospitalization time is shortened.
- Repeated releases are much less.

Section Five

REHABILITATION

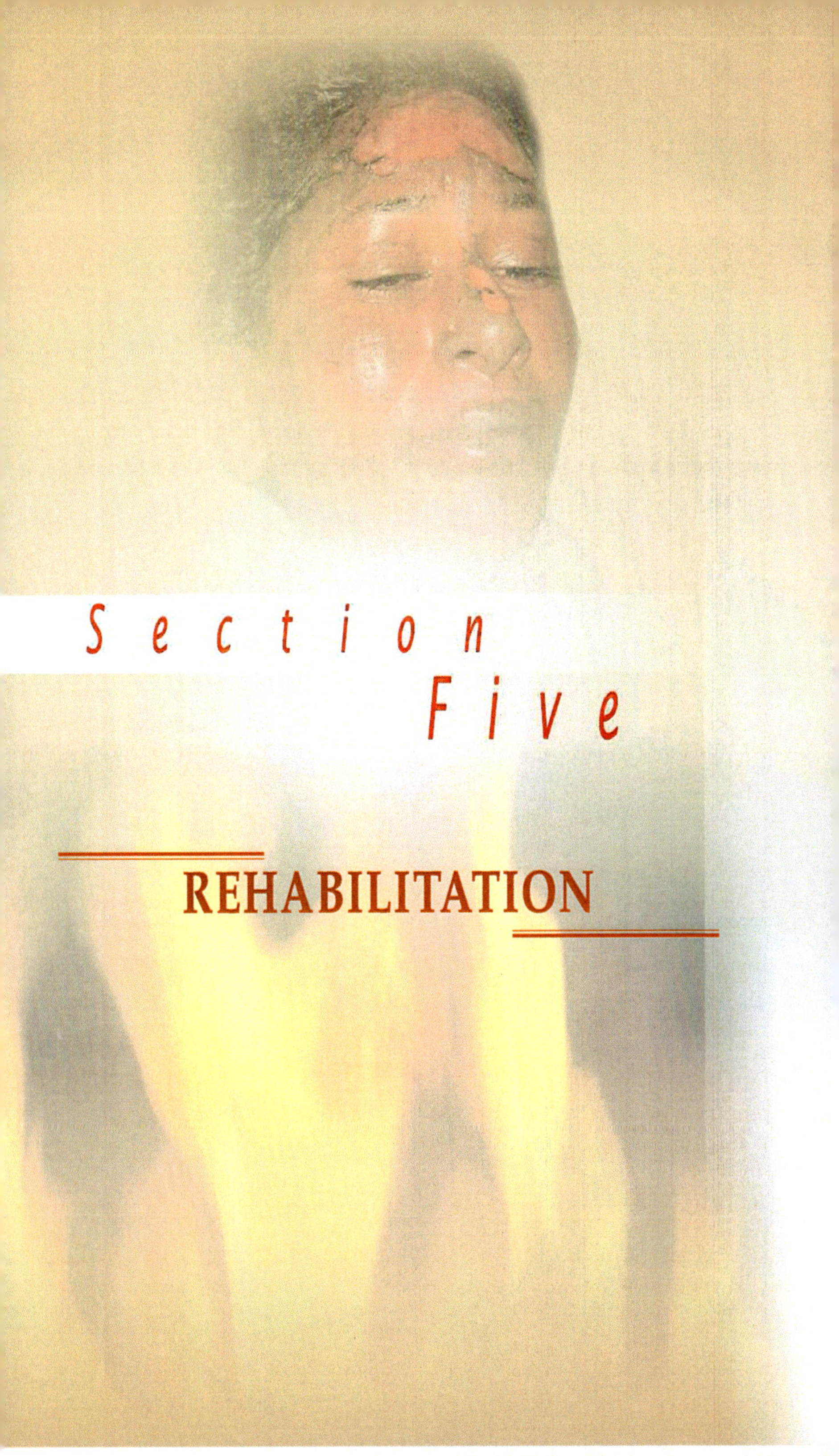

Chapter 31 REHABILITATION PHASE

31.1 INTRODUCTION

- Nursing care of the burn patient is both complex and challenging. The psychological and physical trauma sustained following a burn injury can be devastating for both the victim and family members.Having a thorough understanding of the pathophysiologic changes that occur after a burn and knowing what to expect clinically as a result of the injury, and becoming familiar with the standards of care will guide nursing care to promote positive patient outcomes. Priority issues and care change as the patient moves from the critical emergent phase, recovery phase to rehabilitation phase.
- Rehabilitation is essential for the patients who not only suffer severe burn injury but also undergo mental trauma. The disfigurement that occurs compel them to withdraw from the surrounding. Care is taken to minimize contractures and disfigurement by proper wound care, splinting and physiotherapy.
- The results of burn wound healing and hypertrophic scarring are devastating. Without adequate management patients face a life time of limited motion and functional disabilities, decreased general body strength, unsatisfactory appearance, emotional and social maladjustments.
- Each patient's rehabilitation program must be tailored to his or her specific needs from "post burn day one" throughout recovery until optimal results are achieved and the patient is at maximal functional independence.

- Rehabilitation begins during acute treatment phase and continues to meet each patient's specific needs.
- The goals for helping towards rehabilitation—is to return the patient to highest level of function and independence possible, while improving the overall quality of life physically, emotionally and socially.
- The family members should be involved in dressing, physiotherapy and regular oil message. Patients should be made to realize the importance of self dependency.

31.2 GOALS

- Restore function.
- Prevent contracture.
- Return to normal activities.
- Best aesthetic appearance possible.
- Prevent deformity.
- Protection of the recently healed skin.
- Position the patient opposite to the position of comfort and contracture.

31.3 TECHNIQUES

- Positioning.
- Active range of motion/exercise.
- Pressure therapy.
- Scar management.
- Splinting.
- Activities of daily living.
- Vocational treatment.

Active Range of Motion and Exercise

- Prevent skin contracture.
- Maintain skin joint integrity.
- Prevent muscle atrophy.
- Prevent edema.
- Initiate patient participation.

Examples of Position to Prevent Deformity

Burned area	Position of deformity	Position the patient	Technique
Head and neck	Flexion	Extension or slight hyperextension	• No pillow • Towel roll under shoulder
Wrist and hand	Wrist flexion, MPJt Hyperextension,IP joint flexion	Wrist extension, MP joint flexion IP joint extention	• Arm support • Splint and gauze roll
Knee	Flexion	Extension	• No pillow under leg • Splint

Scar Management/Pressure Therapy

- Control hypertrophic scar.
- Promote healing.
- Assist venous return.

31.4 GARMENTS

They do not prevent contracture. They only flatten scars and aid the normal orientation of collagen fibers.

Pressure Garments

- Garments do not prevent contractures. Exercise/splint/and positioning prevent contractures.
- Hypertrophic scarring is formed when fibroblast produce an excessive amount of collagen fibers which adhere to each other in an irregular pattern.
- Constant and adequate pressure will flatten scars and aid the normal orientation of collagen fibers.

Types of Pressure Garments

Temporary Garments

- Elastic compression bandage should be started when healing is sufficient or may be applied over bandages or can be used after surgeries to protect a graft.
- Pressure must be graduated, highest distally on the extremity and least proximally.

- Patient should wear these garments all times except when bathing.
- Regular care should be taken to monitor areas under garments for increased edema, pressure breakdown of healed skin and increased pain.

Custom made Gradient Pressure Garments

- It is designed to apply 25-30 mm Hg gradient pressure on the scar tissue.
- These garments are expensive and patients must be taught how to properly care for them.
- It should be hand washed, dried flat, evaluated routinely to assure an adequate fit.
- The scarring phase generally begins 3- 4weeks of post burn day and continue for eight to eighteen months.
- Gradient elastic compression is indicated throughout the scar maturation splints process till scar is clinically mature.

Static Splints

These do not allow movement (Figs 31.1 to 31.5)

- Wrist 30 degree extension.
- Metacarpal-phalangeal joint flexion 60-90 degree.
- Interphalangeal joint extension.
- Thumb opposition to prevent claw hand deformity.

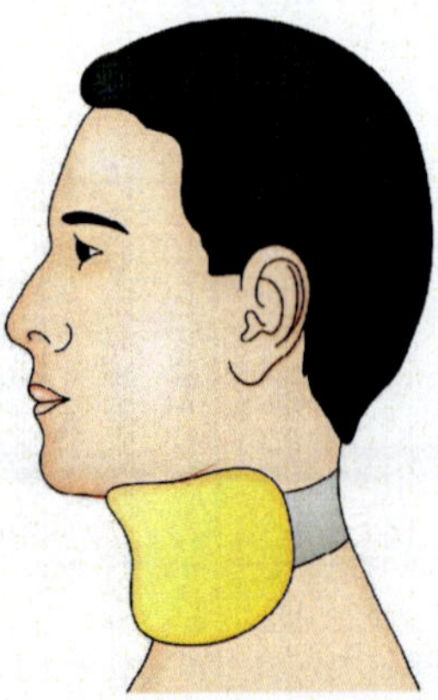

Fig. 31.1: Neck splints should be below the chin

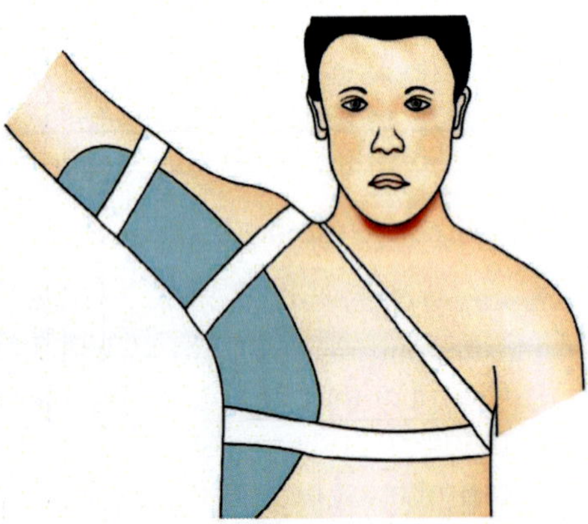

Fig. 31.2: Axillary splint to keep the axilla abducted

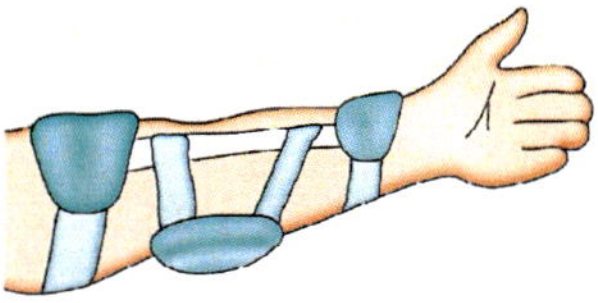

Fig. 31.3: Elbow splint to keep elbow straight

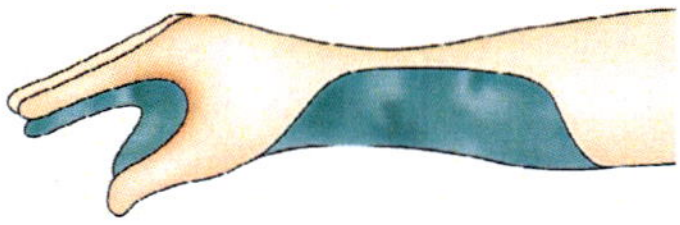

Fig. 31.4: hand splint

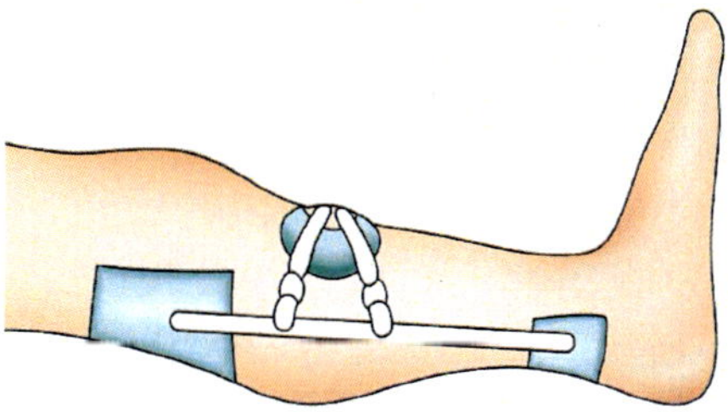

Fig. 31.5: Lower leg splint to keep popliteal region straight

Elbow/Knee Extension Splint (Conformer)

- Prevent and correct flexion contracture.
- Keep the flexor surface of the joint straight.
- Continue until full ROM is regained or graft is adherent.

Neck collar is utilized early to position the head and neck until the wound is nearly healed.

Factors Influencing the Success of Rehabilitation Program

- Coping skill.
- Pain.
- Support system.
- Stress.
- Emotional.
- Environmental.
- Quality of recovery.

Rehabilitation Team

- Doctors
- Nurses
- Psychologists

- Physiotherapist
- Occupational therapist
- Dietician
- Social workers
- Chaplian

In Summary

We know that early splinting and correct positioning of burns can prevent contracture formation, deformity and disability.

Prevention of neck contracture is a challenge for both plastic surgeons and nurses as it causes significant functional restriction. Splinting must commence to maintain length and range of motion in acute stage and through out, until it is healed or grafted. When not suitable for grafting in an acute setting, neck need to be splinted. However, rigid splinting is not practical as the patient needs daily dressing and hence soft collars should be used.

The immediate goals of therapy are to preserve range of motion and function.The long term goals of therapy are to maximize independence in activities of daily living and train the survivors to be as functional as possible despite any loss of extremity.

As soon as the patient is admitted into the burns unit, nurses should position the patient tailored to the patients specific needs. Positioning is important as it decreases the incidence of edema prevents future contractures and deformities. Prevents neurologic trauma , preserves function and promotes wound healing.

31.5 POSITIONING

Head

Burn injury involving the head warrants elevation of the head above the level of the heart to aid in edema reduction. When the patients ear are burned, ear protectors should be used to prevent further injury to the ear cartilage and subsequent chondritis.

The neck should be positioned in neutral to slight extension by keeping a shoulder pillow.

Shoulder

Shoulder should be abducted to 90 degree. Elbow joint positioned in extension.

Wrist and Hand

The wrist should be positioned in up to 30 degree extension. The hand should be positioned with the metacarpophalangeal (MCP) joints between 70-90 degree flexion and the interphalangeal joints (IP) in extension. This position will prevent tightness of the collateral ligaments that fold around the volar plates and future stiffness of the active hand. The thumb IP and MCP joints should be positioned in a combined radial and palmar abduction thus preventing a cupping contracture of the palm.

Hip

The hips should be positioned in extension . In 0-15 degree abduction, pillows or foam wedges can be placed between the thighs

Knee

The knees should be positioned in extension.

Ankle and Foot

The ankle joint should be positioned at 90 degree in relation to the rest of the lower extremity. Corrective surgeries for postburn deformities with hypertrophic scarring and contractures are demanding and hence prevention should be the goal.

Splinting

Patients with severe burns are at risk for development of limited joint mobility. A splint program for contracture management includes both active and passive mobilization . Splints are used to counteract the initial and ongoing contraction of wounded tissue to the time of scar maturation.

Casting

Serial casting can be a tremendous adjunct to a therapeutic exercise program for rehabilitation after burn injury. When the use of passive range of motion positioning and splinting have failed to correct burn contractures , serial casting can be effective in helping to increase the range of motion.

Prosthetics

Burn injuries can require amputation because of the depth of burn injury. The use of prosthetics greatly aides in the restoration of function to patients who have sustained amputations.

Scar Management

As the burn wound heals it forms scar tissue at the site of injury characterized by abundance of collagen fibers. Scar hypertrophy may be evident at 12 weeks after the injury. The newly formed scar seems to be red, raised and rigid and is known as immature scar. This scar responds to pressure therapy. Burn scars are treated by means of pressure therapy, application of physical agent modalities, massage and exercise.

Pressure Therapy

Pressure causes devascularization. Decreased blood flow to the scar leads to decreased production of collagen fibers causing a balance in the synthesis and breakdown of collagen, such a balance produces a flatter, softer and less vascularized scar. Pressure garments should be worn on a 24 hour basis. Initially the pressure applied should be low (10-15 mm of Hg). Low pressure garments include tubular bandages and elastocrepe bandages. As the burn scar progresses in the maturation process custom made pressure garments providing 24-28 mm of Hg should be used.

Inserts

Various insert materials may be used beneath pressure garments such as foam and silicon gel.

Massage

This helps to soften the scar and should be a part of a home exercise program.

31.6 CONCLUSION

Success is Achieved Through

- Commitment
- Team spirit
- Co-operation of patient, family and society.

Chapter

32 REHABILITATION OF HAND BURNS

32.1 INTRODUCTION

Burns of the hand is a crippling problem. It occurs both as an isolated injury or a part of the major burn injury.

Function

- It is a means of expression.
- A receptor of sensory information.
- A tool necessary for performing functional activity.

Thermal injury is one of the most devastating physical and psycho logical injuries a person can suffer if appropriate treatment is not received in a timely manner.

- Caused by thermal, chemical and electrical.
- Problem in all types of burn is loss of skin.
- Palmar surface burns—thick skin, so problems are less.
- Dorsal burns—thin skin, burns is deeper and contractures are common.

Prevention of Deformity

- Immediate rehabilitative intervention.
- Proper positioning with splints.
- Exercise to maintain range of motion in joints.
- Maintenance of muscle strength and muscle tone.
- Early mobilization.

Pathology of Hand Burns

- Following burns -Increased capillary permeability.

- Out pouring of protein rich fluid which soaks collateral ligament of small joints.
- Connective tissue around tendons.
- Broad expansion of extensor mechanism.
- Collagen synthesis and remodeling causes stiff joints.

Contributing Factors

- Edema.
- Wound infection.
- Poor positioning.
- Prolonged immobilization.
- Delayed skin cover.

Aim of Treatment (Figs 32.1 and 32.2)

- Reduce edema and maintain range of movement.
- Prevent deformity by positioning and splinting.
- Minimize scarring by using pressure techniques.
- Improve muscle strength.

Three Phases of Rehabilitation

- Acute care.
- Surgical and post operative period.
- Rehabilitation of out patient - (Most challenging phase of all).

Role of Therapist

- Acute care – prevention
- Surgical and post op – Assist surgeon to preserve function
- Rehabilitative phase – control scar maturation
- Prevent deformity and contracture.

Management of Burned Hand

- Represents a fascinating concept of wound healing.
- Multiple techniques are available with superior results.
- The challenges have peaked.
- Results have steadily improved.
- Choice of correct modality of treatment remains the greatest challenge.

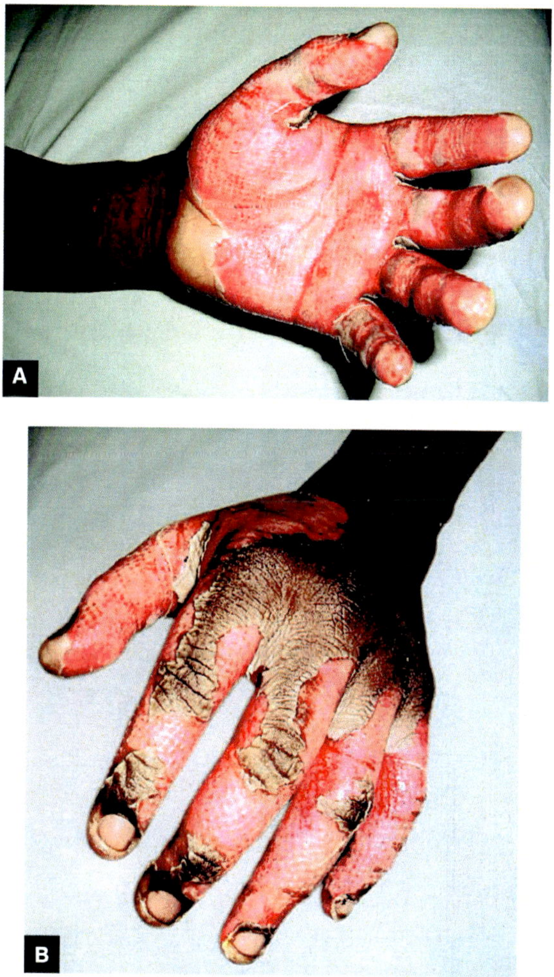

Figs 32.1 A and B: Acute burns-hydrotherapy treatment

Timing of Reconstruction

- **Early (scars immature):** Progressive deformity and progressive functional deficit.
- **Late (scars mature):** No progressive functional deficit, deformities stable.
- Although medical issues are a primary concern.

- There is no substitute for early and consistent intervention by therapist.

Classification of Burn Deformity

Soft tissue deformity:
- Palmar contracture (Figs 32.3 and 32.4).
- Dorsal contracture (Figs 32.5 and 32.6).
- Web space contracture (Figs 32.7 to 32.9).
- Adduction contracture
- Hypertrophic scar

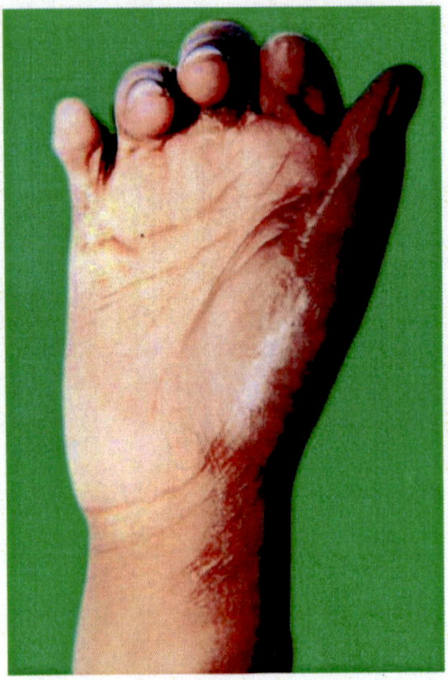

Fig. 32.3: Flexion contracture of hand

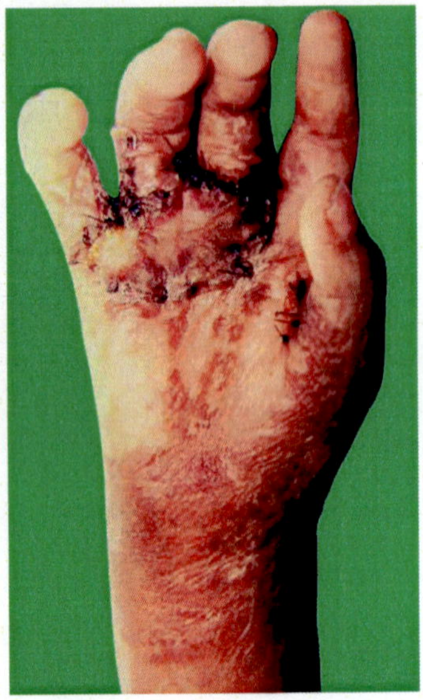

Fig. 32.4: Contracture release with graft from the sole

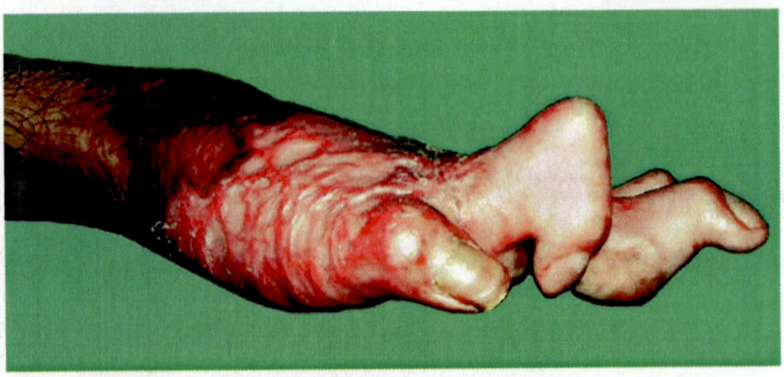

Fig. 32.5: Contracture of hand

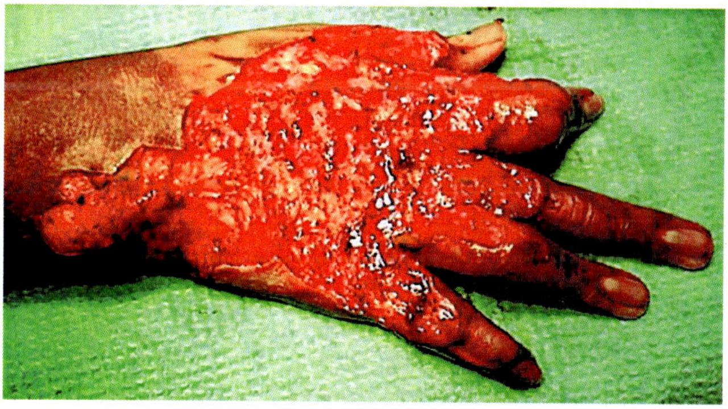

Fig. 32.6: Dorsal contracture release

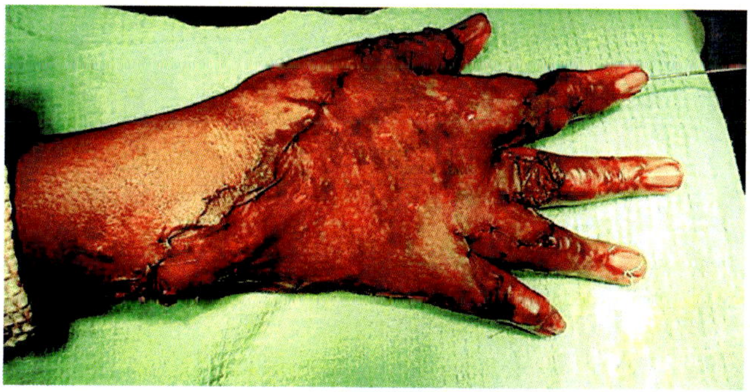

Fig. 32.7: Dorsal contracture release with graft

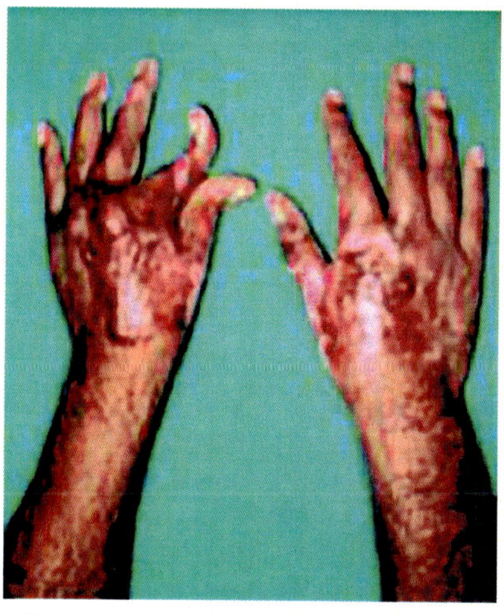

Fig. 32.8: First web space contracture

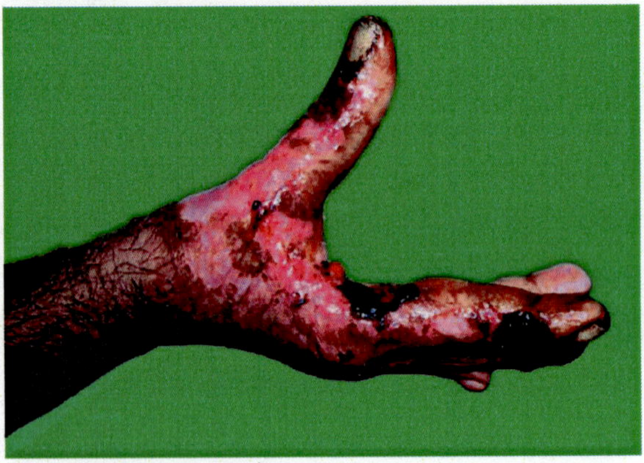

Fig. 32.9: Four flap release of first web space

Joint deformity:

- MCP (claw)
- PIP (boutonniere)
- DIP (mallet) (Figs. 32.10 to 32.13)
- Nail deformity
- Amputation
- Complex deformity

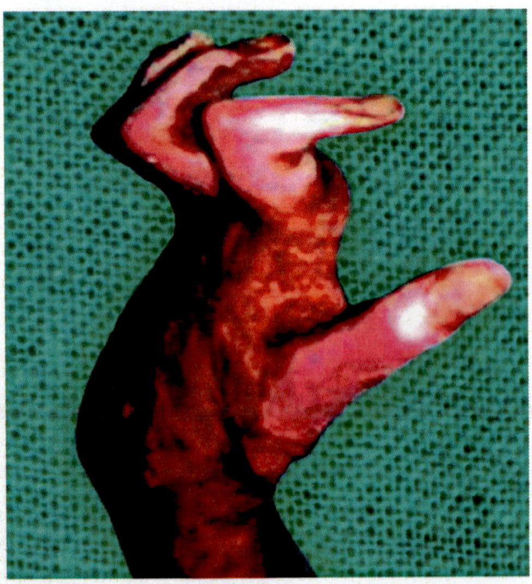

Fig. 32.10: MP extension and IP flexion contracture

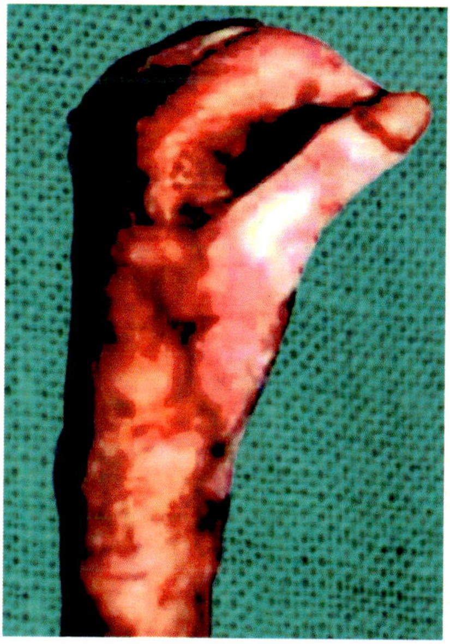

Fig. 32.11: Post MP and IP correction

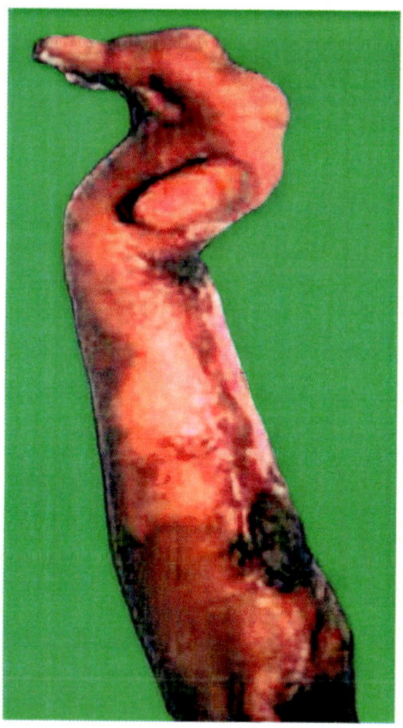

Fig. 32.12: Hyperextension contracture

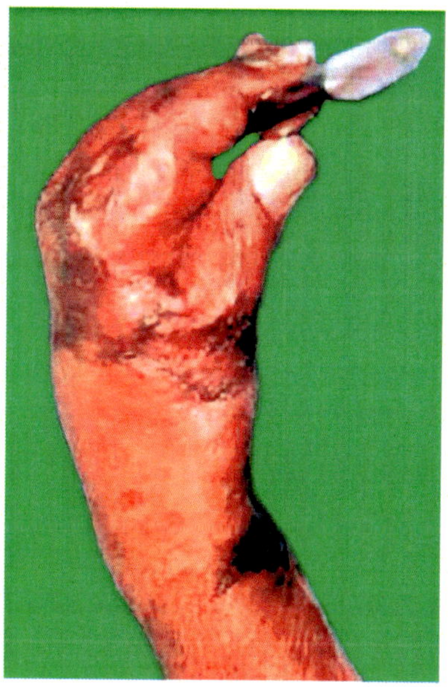

Fig. 32.13: Posthyperextension deformity correction

Post Burn Claw Hand

- Typical deformity resulting from unopposed contracture from a dorsal hand burn.
- Hyperextension at the metacarpo-phalangeal joints.
- Flexion at the proximal interphalangeal joints.

Boutonniere

- Deeply burned PIP joint.
- Destruction of the central slip of the extensor tendon over the PIP Joint.

Swan Neck Deformity

- MCP Joint flexion.
- PIP Joint hyperextension.
- DIP Joint flexion.

Role of Occupational and Physiotherapy

- To use a variety of therapeutic interventions in order to promote a return to maximum independent living.
- Primary requisite is surgical release of contractures followed by
    - Heat,
    - Active and passive motion.
    - Dynamic and static splints.

Advantages of Pressure Therapy

- Reduce edema.
- Diminishes discomfort.
- Prevents itching.
- Scar matures.

Maintenance of Function

- Rehabilitation therapy upon admission.
- Continued through out hospitalization.
- Maintained postoperatively for a period of two years or more.

32.2 CONCLUSION

- Physical and occupational therapist have professional skills, equipments, technology and resources undreamed of just a few years ago.

- Therapists make critical contributions to the achievement of successful rehabilitation outcomes.
- Occupational therapist form an integral part of the burn team-by preventing soft tissue contractures, which are the major cause of loss of function and distortion.

32.3 ROLE OF NURSES

Your continued efforts will go a long way to help burn victims to be independent and return to society as close as possible to their pre-injury level of function.

Chapter

33 MAKE UP FOR BURN PATIENTS

The survival rate following extensive burns have increased. The reconstructive techniques have significantly altered the appearance by using the various non surgical and surgical methods, but still there are limitations to surgical intervention. It is here that make up cream helps the patient to face the society with confidence.

Non-Surgical

- Pressure garments
- Splinting
- Silicone conformers
- Moisturizing lotion.

Surgical

- Scar excision
- Skin grafts
- Local flaps
- Tissue expansion
- Free flaps.

Goals of make up

- Minimize the psychological impact of burn injury
- Promote social rehabilitation
- Minimize visible scars

Cosmetic camouflage (Figs 33.1 to 33.7).

- Application of make up conceals scars and pigmentation changes
- Has no gender or racial limitation
- Hypopigmented scars are camouflaged with concealing creams

- Hyperpigmented skin grafts can also be treated by using bleaching creams.

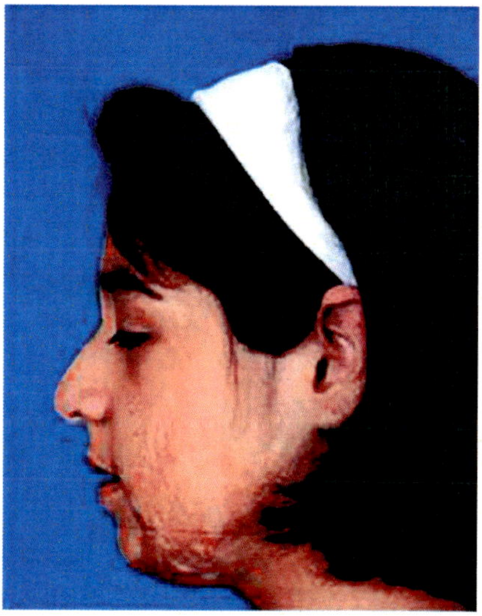

Fig. 33.1: Burns of face

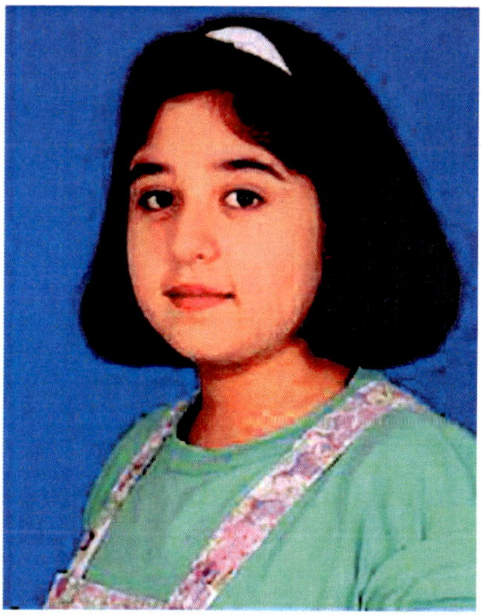

Figs. 33.2: After cosmetic cream

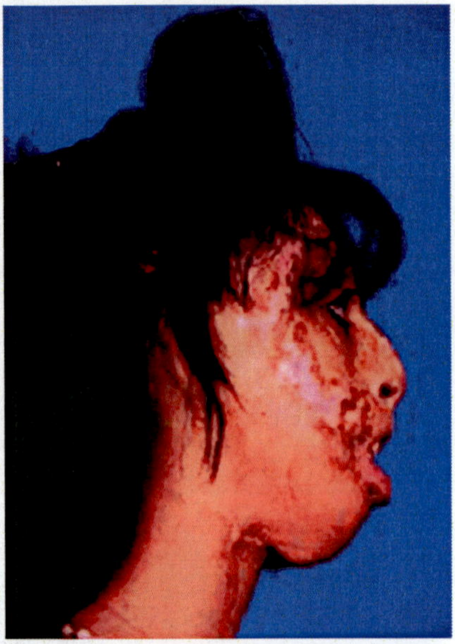

Fig. 33.3: Hyper and hypopigmentation

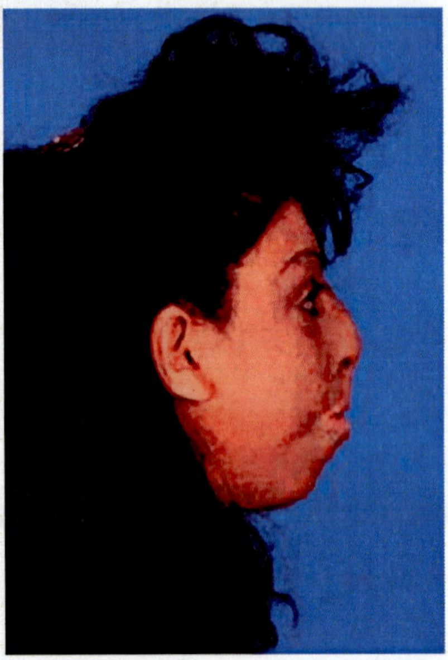

Fig. 33.4: Camouflage of both pigmentation

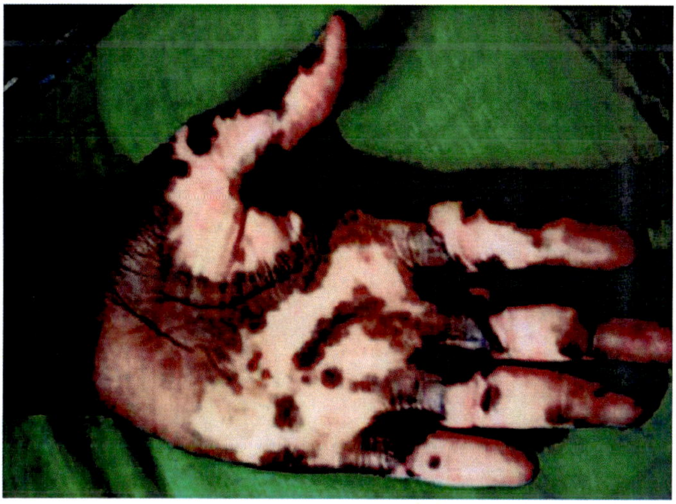

Fig. 33.5: Burns hand

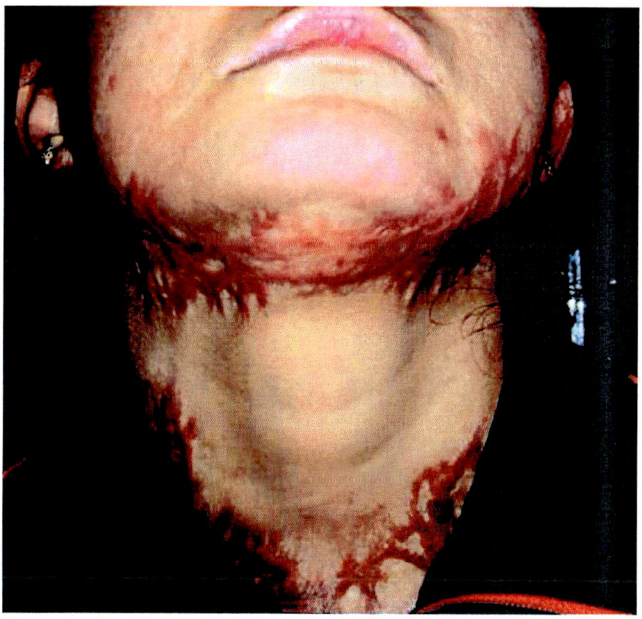

Fig. 33.6: Hypertrophic scar

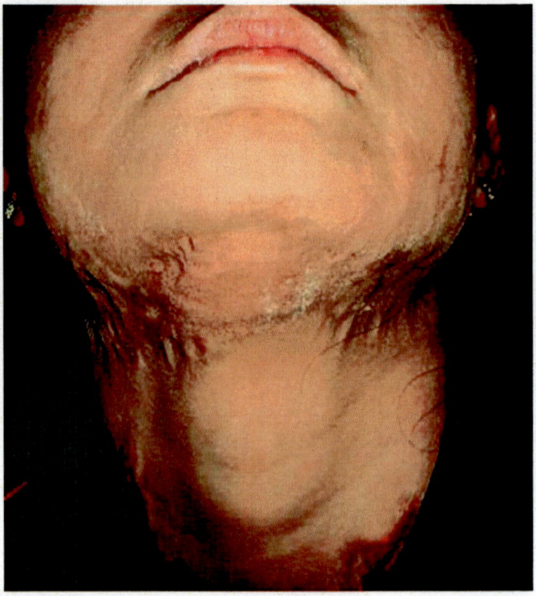

Fig. 33.7: After camouflage

Types of Make Up

- Foundation
- Corrective cosmetics
    - Setting powder
    - Compact powder
- Regular cosmetics.

Benefits

- Restores confidence and self image.
- Survivors reintegrated into society.
- Reintegration into society is a testimony to the beneficial effects of cosmetics on improving the psychological outlook of patients.

Conclusion

- Cosmetics is a useful adjunct to surgical intervention.
- Lessens the impact of visible scars and pigmentation differences.
- Enhances self image and confidence.

Chapter

34 PSYCHOLOGICAL SUPPORT OF BURN SURVIVORS

Many people get afflicted with burns either by accident or injury. These survivors experience great physical and psychological trauma.

Many burn survivors , fear being rejected and sometimes begin to hide themselves in a world of their own. Integrating back into society is difficult, and for many being accepted by their own family members is a struggle.

At the time of injury every burns victim needs support, encouragement and guidance for accepting his or her disability.

The extent of physical, emotional and psychological trauma is dependent upon a number of factors, these include the kind of burns inflicted, visibility and the invisibility of the disfigurement, the way the patient gets burnt (accidental, inflicted by self, caused by others) and the age of the individual. It is necessary that the burn survivors be supported in accepting their new body image.

Most important of all burn survivors must be assisted to discover, recognize and affirm their strengths and focus upon them. One method of help is to increase sense of self- worth is through the organization of self-help groups. These are informal groups run by members who share a common illness or handicap.

Self help groups provide the patients the experience of knowing that they are not alone in their struggle. This helps them ventilate their feeling of fear, anger and loneliness in a non threatening atmosphere and helps provide them the opportunity to learn practical coping skills from the positive role models (i.e. those who have survived accepted and are coping effectively despite their disability illness).

Families and spouses of the burn survivors also need support and guidance and they can also be included in the self-help groups. In some cases it becomes necessary to provide them individual counseling to enable them to get over their psychological trauma and to regain their emotional strength to face life effectively.

It is necessary to approach the pain and suffering of burn survivors with sensitivity and strength. A great deal of emotional support must be provided to help them to alleviate their fears, anxieties and doubts throughout the rehabilitation period. Therefore one of the primary humanitarian duty of every individual is to help the burn survivors to have hope and faith in the future and to make them realize the gracious gift of a second life.

34.1 PROBLEMS

- Patients feel that they are separated from family and friends.
- A feeling of rejection sets in.
- They undergo fear, anxiety and depression because they are depended on others for their daily activities.

34.2 ROLE OF NURSES IN EMOTIONAL SUPPORT

- Emotional support through counseling will encourage the patient to have a positive look towards early recovery.
- Patients should be involved in activities and develop confidence in the medical staff.
- The family and friends should be made to give total support and encouragement to the patient.
- Frequent visits by family should be encouraged so that the family starts accepting the disfigurement and disability.
- Referring the patient and family to the self help groups.

Chapter

35 BURN UNIT

The concept of specialized burn unit was started in the USA some 50 years ago and much later in India. Along with it the importance was also given to medical technology provided by multispeciality and multidisciplinary teams.

Burn unit is a specialized area within the hospital. It has a specialized nursing team dedicated to burn patient care.

Burn unit should be part of a teaching hospital with ICU facility. It should be staffed by a team of professionals with expertise in the care of burn patients and includes both acute care, reconstruction and rehabilitation.

A burn team should also provide educational programs regarding burn care to all health care providers and involve in research related to burn injury.

The cost of running a burn unit is enormous. The over all design of burns unit will depend on the required size and available finance. The principles of prevention of infection in the burn unit are more important than airborne spread.

Hand washing is therefore more important than complex air conditioning (wash basin in each patient's room). Well ventilated single rooms with ICU standards is preferable. Burn nurses in uniform, caps, masks and rubber slippers to be used only in the burn unit. Relatives should be provided with gowns, masks, caps and overshoes before entering the burn unit.

Sterile linen to be changed every day. Thorough cleaning of the rooms every day with 4% lysol.

When the patient is discharged the rooms are cleaned for three consecutive days with soap and water followed by 4% Lysol. This procedure has proved to be adequate and has replaced the old tedious fumigation procedure.

Once a year the whole burn unit is closed for thorough cleaning.

Chapter

36 PREVENTION OF BURNS

36.1 INTRODUCTION

- Burn injuries are universal.
- Incidence is on the increase with the complexities of modern living and industrialization,
- Most of the burns occur either at home or at the place of work, and hence it becomes important to know about burns.

Q. What causes burns?

Ans. Burns can be caused by flame, acid, hot liquids and electricity.

Q. What to do immediately following burns?

Ans. Priority is to stop the burning process by using tap water.

Q. Can water cause blisters?

Ans. No. Blisters indicates that burns are superficial and will heal spontaneously.

Q. What to apply on the burnt surface?

Ans. Apply ointments like neosporin, soframycin, silver sulfa diazine. Do not apply gention violet, ink, ghee, calamine, lotion, salt, tooth paste, etc.

Do's

- Pour water to stop the burning process (Fig. 36.1).
- If no water, stop, drop and roll

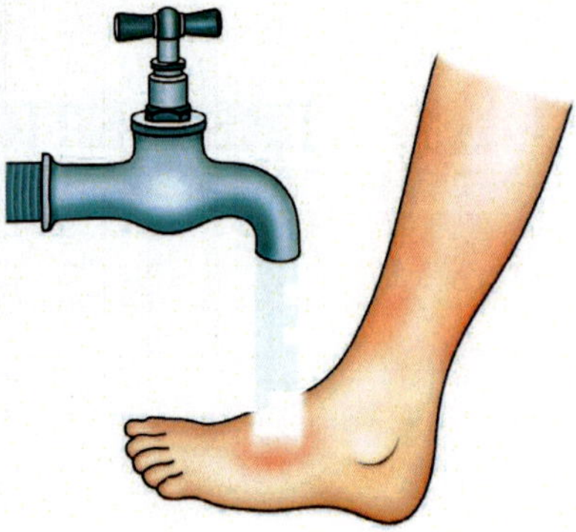

Fig. 36.1: Pour water on burns till pain stops

Dont 's

- Do not play with matches, kerosene, fire cracker and electricity (Figs 36.2 to 36.4).
- Do not pour kerosene or petrol to revive fire (Fig. 36.5)
- Do not cook on a large flame (Fig. 36.6)
- Do not leave gas inlet open when not in use (Figs 36.7)
- Do not keep cylinder near electrical socket (Fig. 36.8)
- If gas leak is suspected in the kitchen do not strike a match or put the electric switch on, or smoke. Open the windows and tighten all gas valves. If it is still leaking call gas company
- Do not use loose pressure cooker rubber (casket) (Fig. 36.9)
- Do not carry hot water on a slippery floor
- Never leave a child unattended in the bathroom
- Do not keep open fire near the bed on a winter night
- When you go on long leave, disconnect the plug of radio, television and other electrical appliances
- Do not allow children near hot silencer
- Do not keep the test tube close to your face in chemistry lab. Use adequate protection (Fig. 36.10).

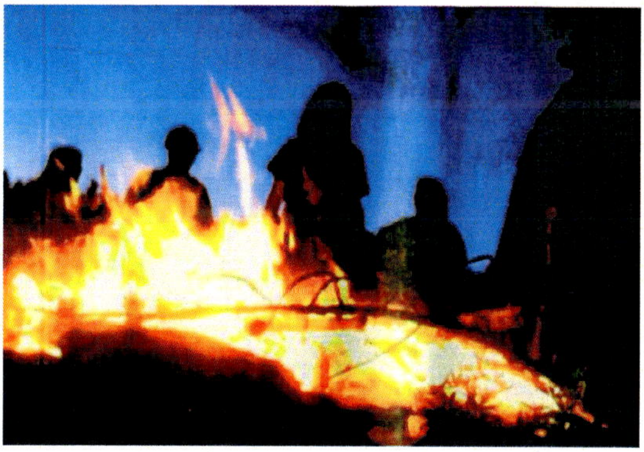

Fig. 36.2: Do not play with fire

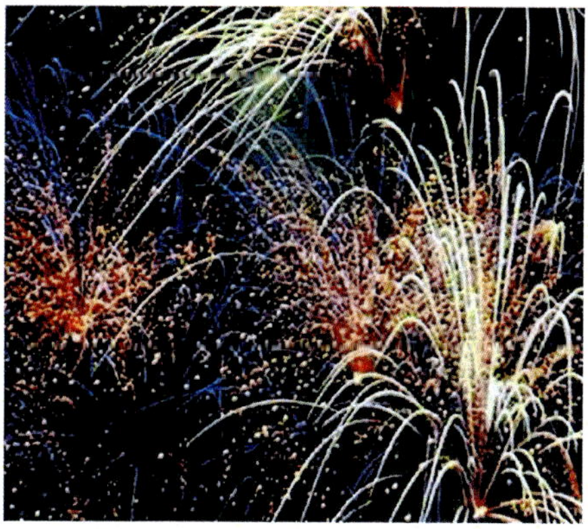

Fig. 36.3: Do not play with firecracker

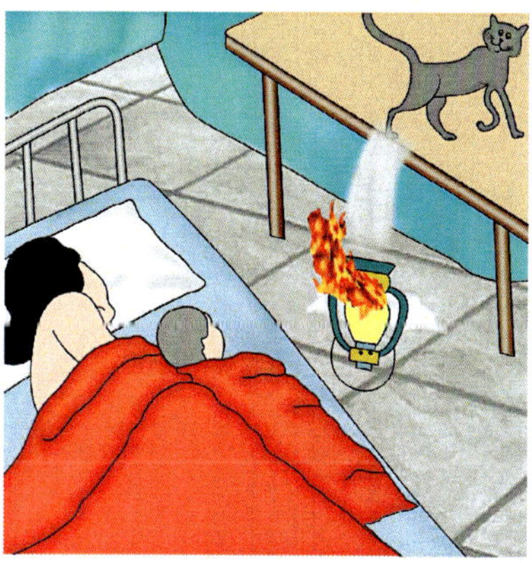

Fig. 36.4: Do not keep kerosine lamp near the bed

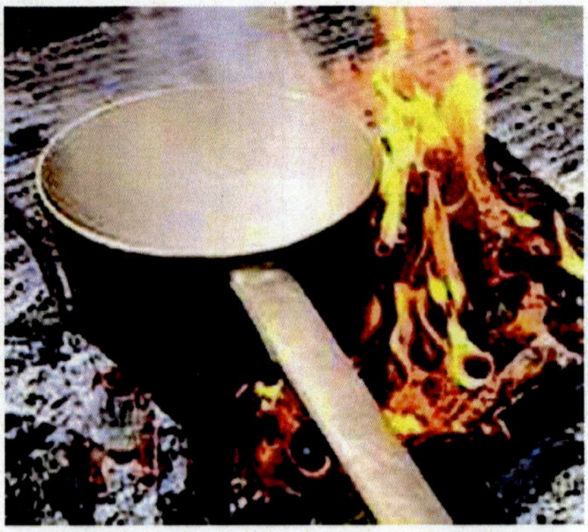

Fig. 36.5: Do not pour kerosine to increase the flame

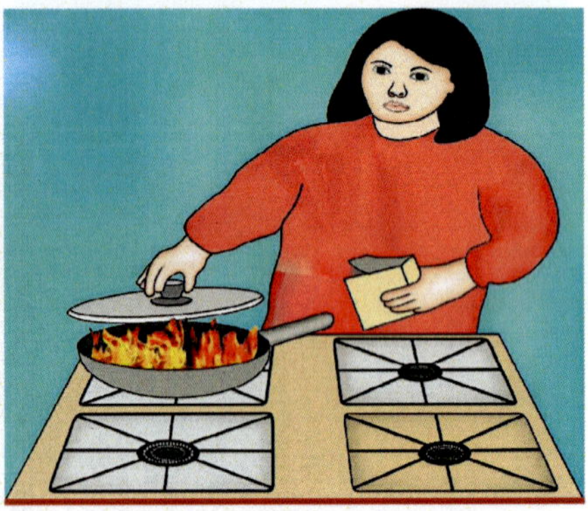

Fig. 36.6: Do not cook under huge flame

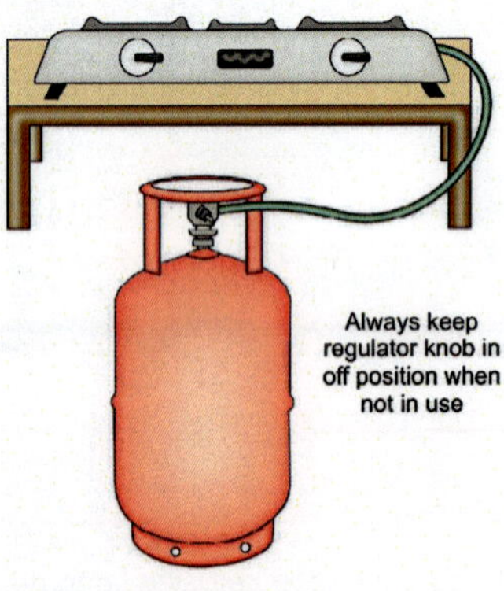

Fig. 36.7: Gas inlet should be closed when not in use

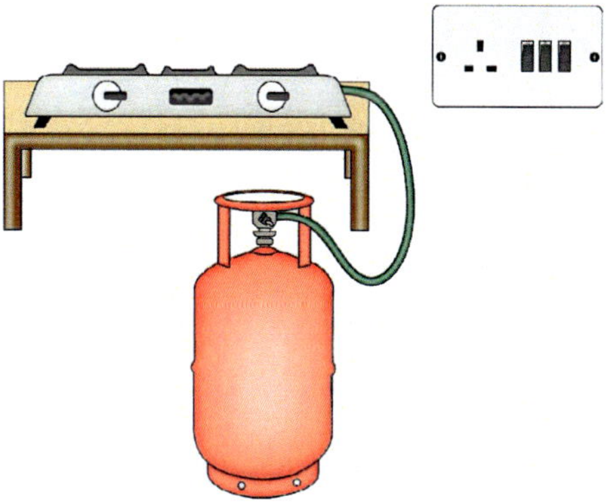

Fig. 36.8: Avoid Keeping gas cylinder near electrical appliances turn of cylinder value first

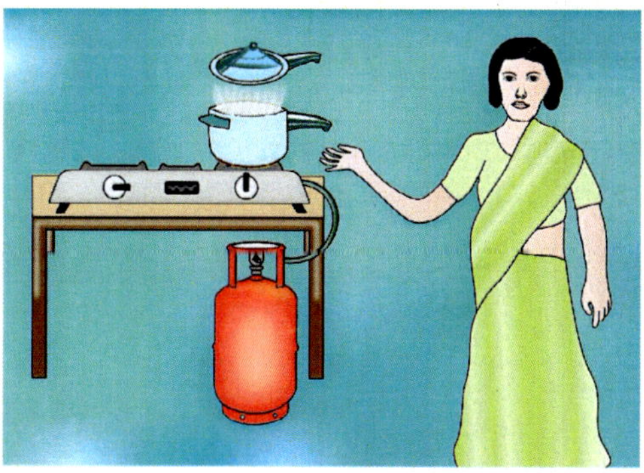

Fig. 36.9: Do not use loose pressure cooker rubber

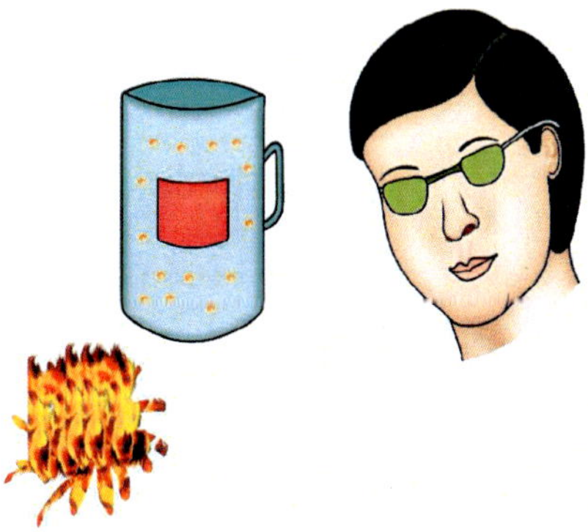

Fig. 36.10: Use adequate protection to prevent industrial flash bums

Avoid

- Avoid cooking on floor level (Fig. 36.11)
- Avoid leaving unattended hot liquids.
- Avoid children playing in the kitchen (Figs 36.12 to 36.14).
- Avoid wearing loose garments in the kitchen (Fig. 36.15).
- Avoid storing cooking materials across the stove
- Avoid using sari to handle vessels (Fig. 36.16)
- Avoid bending over the flame to put out fire (Fig.36.17 and 36.18)
- Avoid keeping stove/candle near gas cylinder.
- Avoid carrying hot things while children are around.
- Avoid keeping mosquito coil near the bed.
- Avoid open plug point (Fig. 36.19).
- Avoid live wires (Figs 36.20 and 36.21).
- Avoid open bathrooms if immersion rod is used to heat water. (Fig. 36.22)
- Avoid using one plug point for many gagets at the same time (Fig. 36.23).

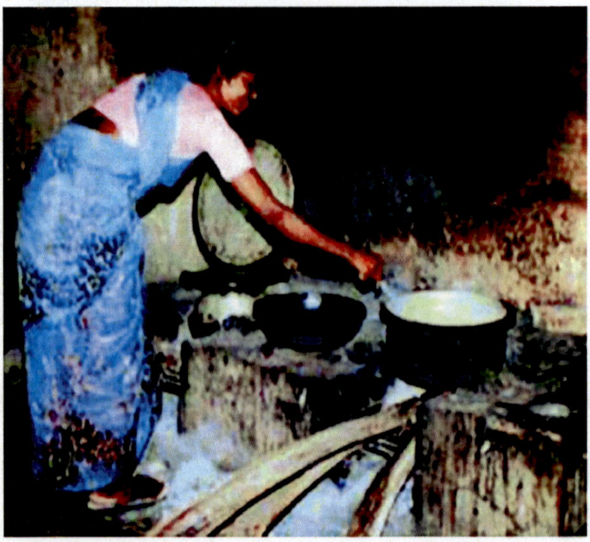

Fig. 36.11: Avoid cooking on floor level

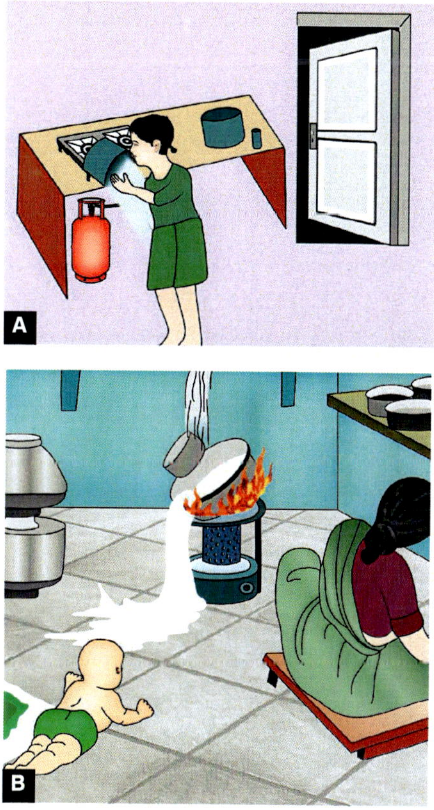

Figs 36.12 A and B: Avoid children in the kitchen

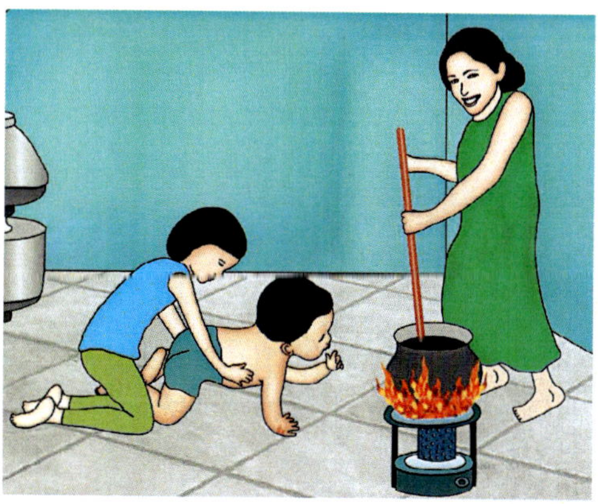

Fig. 36.13: Avoid children playing in the kitchen

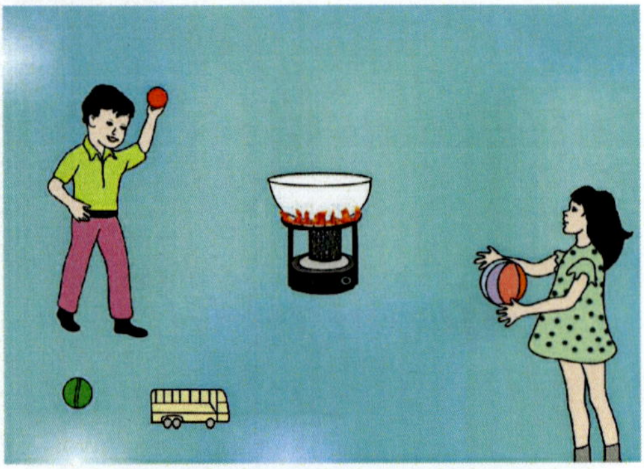

Fig. 36.14: Do not allow the children to play in the kitchen

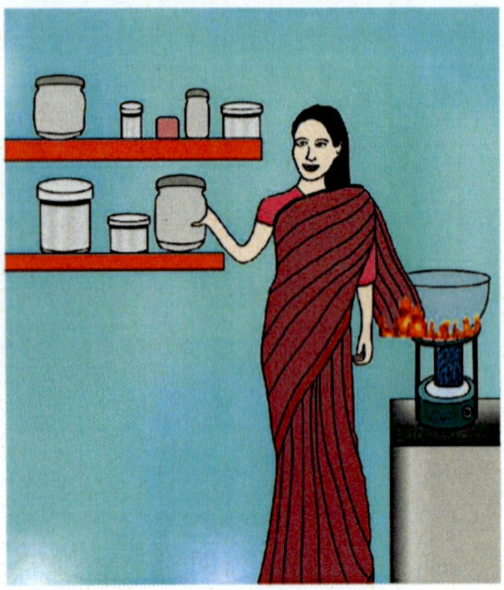

Fig. 36.15: Do not wear loose garment in the kitchen

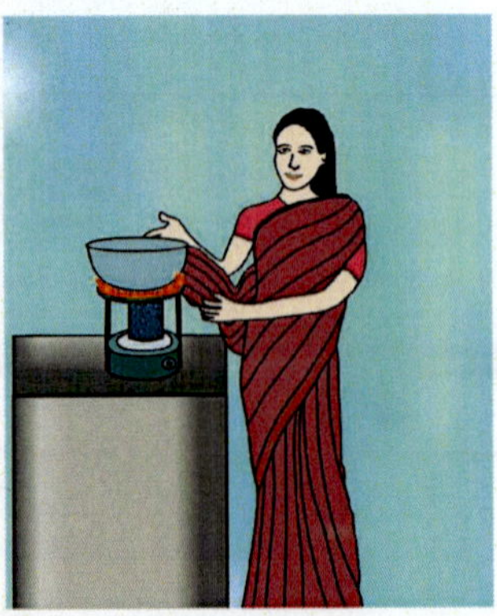

Fig. 36.16: Do not use saree to hold hot vessel

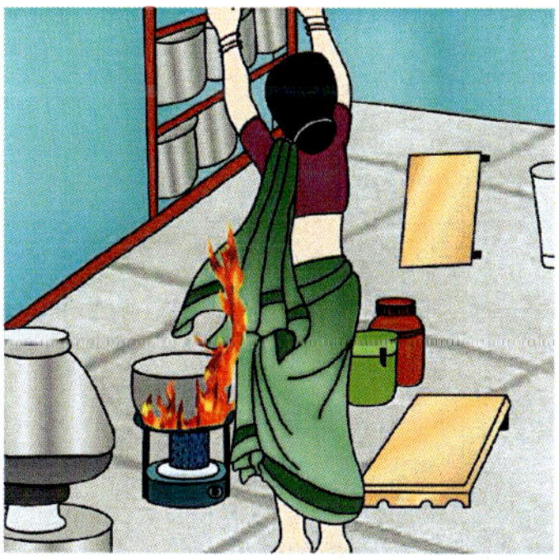

Fig. 36.17: Avoid bending over the flame

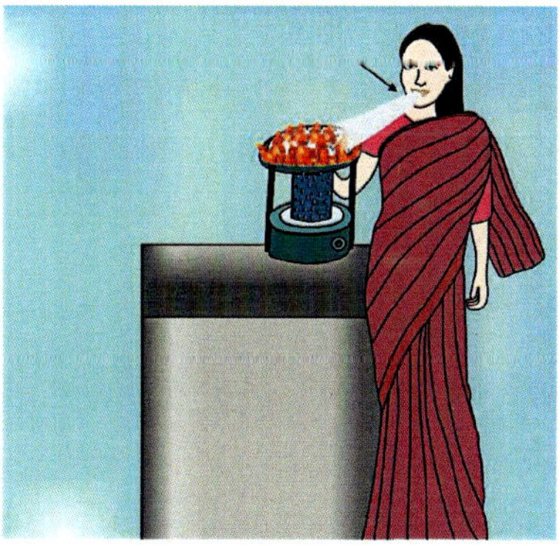

Fig. 36.18: Do not bend and blow the fire

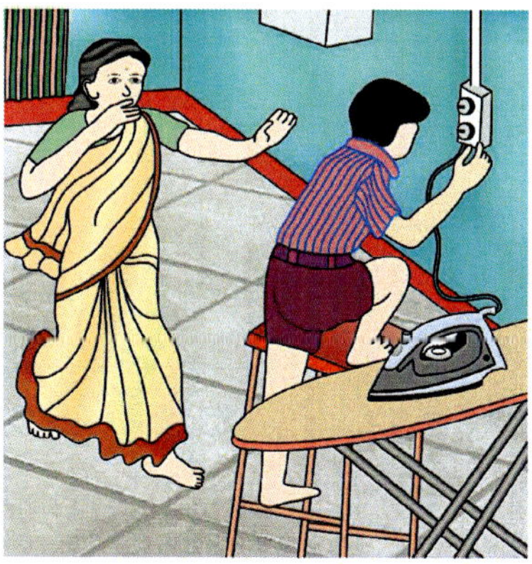

Fig. 36.19: Avoid open plug point

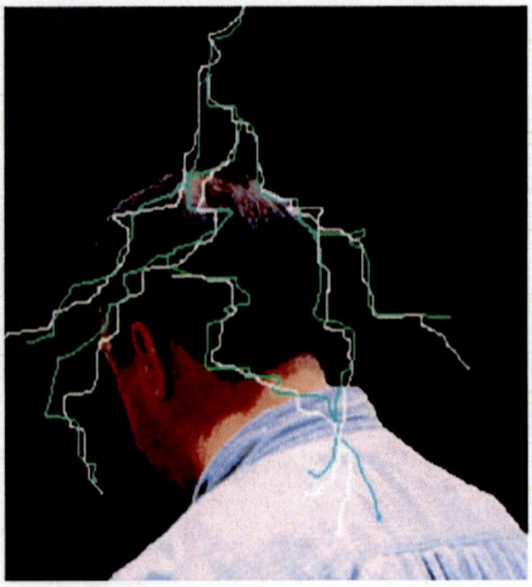

Fig. 36.20: Avoid live wires

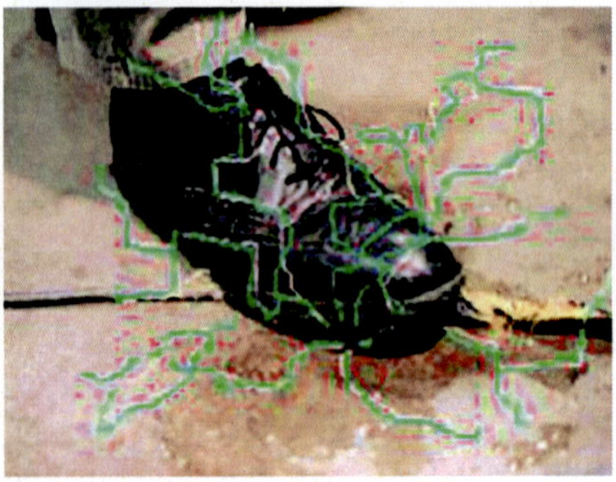

Fig. 36.21: Do not stamp live wires

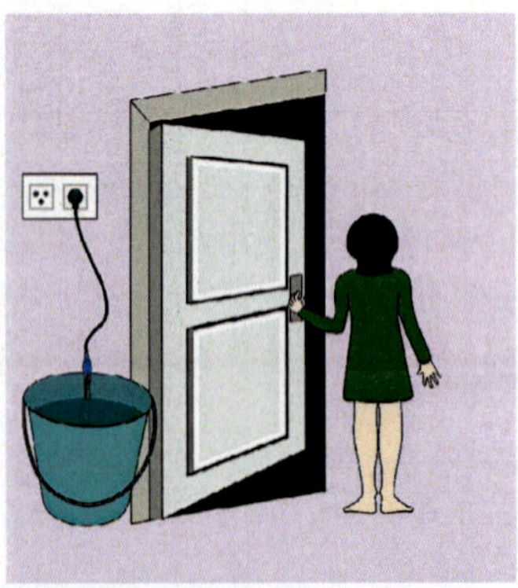

Fig. 36.22: Bathroom door should always be kept closed when immersion rod is used for heating water

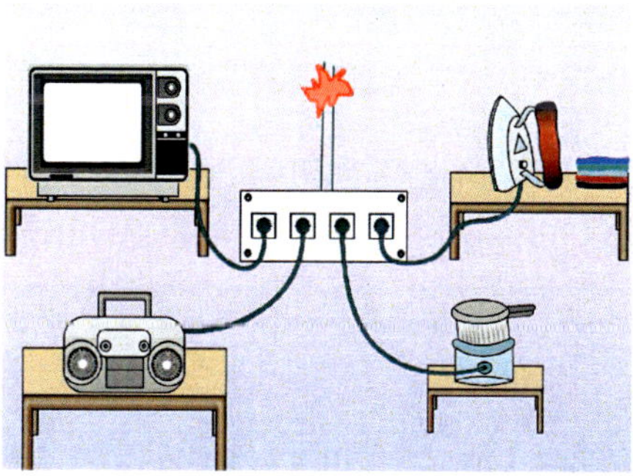

Fig. 36.23: Avoid using one plug point for multiple gaggets

Smoking

- Do not smoke in bed (Fig. 36.24)
- Do not throw matches/cigarette butts carelessly.
- Do not smoke near flammable liquid or gases.

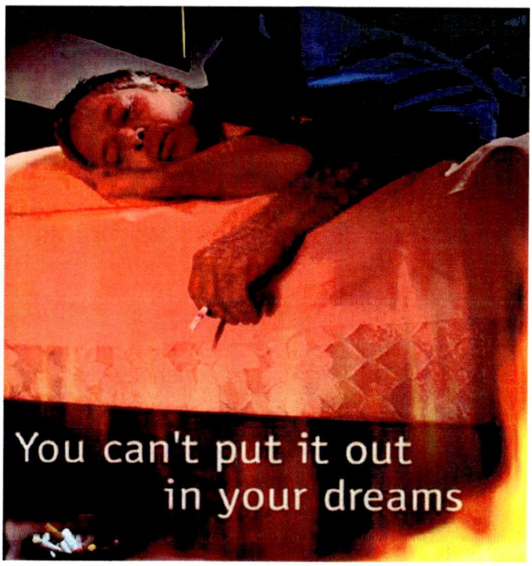

Fig. 36.24: Do not smoke in bed

Flame Burns

- Remove the victim from the site of fire.
- Pour water to cool the burning process.

- Do not allow them to run as this adds oxygen to fire and increases the flame.
- Flames are either put out by water or smothered by rolling on the ground or wrapping in a blanket which is removed as soon as the fire is put out because it tends to retain heat.

Scald Burns

Hot water, milk, tea, oil spilling accidentally are the common causes of burns in Indian kitchen. Hot liquid burns are very common in children and is due to knocking of hot liquid onto them or by stumbling onto a burning agent.

How to Avoid

Keep children away from the kitchen, avoid using tablecloth.

Treatment

Soaked clothes should be immediately removed and cold water poured over the injured areas, apply ointments like Neosporin.

Acid Burns

Acid burns occur in laboratories and at home. They cause full thickness burns. Immediate first aid management is by removing the clothes and washing the burned area with copious amount of water.

(At least 20-30 minutes of washing is necessary to dilute the chemicals). Take the patient to the hospital immediately.

Electrical Burns

The rescuer must be careful so that he does not become a part of the electrical circuit in attempting to free a person still in contact with a live wire.

Use dry wood and push the patient away from current source. Keep the electric wire away from the child as they may bite the live wire. Take the patient to a hospital.

Burns Due to Fire Crackers

Causes serious injury to the eyes, face and hand. Fire works during festivals should be performed in the presence of adults.

During blast injuries sand or gunpowder particles may get impregnated into the skin, so thorough cleaning of the wound is mandatory.

Car Fire

Engine Burning?

- Turn off ignition.
- Do not pour water in an empty hot car radiator, wait to cool or keep the face away from the radiator while pouring water (Fig. 36.25).

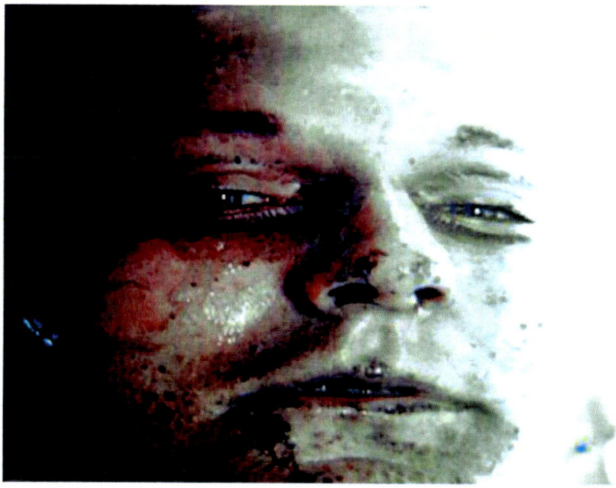

Fig. 36.25 : Prevention of Burns

General Measures

- Once the patient is burnt.
- Put off the fire.
- Remove clothes.
- Wrap in dry cloth.
- Take the patient to the hospital.
  (Please note speed is not necessary in burns).

Prevention of Deformities in Burn Patients

- Proper positioning with splints.
- Regular exercise to maintain motion in joints.
- Early mobilization.

Physiotherapy

- It plays a major role in the management of burn patients. To achieve a functional result continuous effort by the nurse in the burn unit is essential.
- The important aspect is chest physiotherapy and breathing exercises.
- Positioning of the patient—burns can cause permanent deformity and disability. The best way to prevent this is to keep the patient mobile by active and passive exercise starting at the time of admission.

Appropriate Positioning in the Bed

- Supine position.
- Neck in slight extension.
- Arms elevated and abducted.
- Elbows in extension.
- Hand - wrist in 15 degree extension.
  - MP 90 degree flexion.
  - IP extension.
  - Thumb abducted and apposed.
- Hip extended and abducted.
- Knee extended.
- Foot in neutral position or dorsiflexion.

Pressure for Scar Management

Helps to – Reduce edema,
– Reduce discomfort
– Reduce itching
– Scar maturation

Methods of pressure – Elastocrepe bandage
– Coban particularly during the acute period
– Jobst custom pressure garment
– Silicone gel sheet
– Contratubex ointment.

Prevention

- Burn prevention is the best burn care,
- Burn injuries are physically and emotionally devastating.
- It is a financial nightmare for families and hospitals.
- Most of the burns can be prevented.
- It is our responsibility to inform the community about burn prevention.

Preventive Program

- Spreading knowledge.
- Improving quality of burn care.
- Rehabilitation.
- Prevention by organizing seminars.
- Publication of articles in journals and newspaper.
- Display of hoardings at public places.
- Talks in television and school education program are all important tool for awareness program.

36.2 CONCLUSION

- At all stages there is a need for prevention
- Firstly prevention of injury itself -Programmes
- Secondly prevention of infection
- Thirdly decreasing mortality by preventing infection and careful attention to nutrition
- Fourthly prevention of deformity and disability by regular physiotherapy/splinting

36.3 GOALS OF THE NURSE

- Update the knowledge.
- Observe carefully for change in patients condition.
- Be prompt in reporting.
- Develop good rapport with patients relatives and team members.

Chapter

37 BURNS: THE INDIAN SCENARIO

The Challenge that is Cultural, Social Economic and Political

India is a vast land with many religions and diverse customs. The strong religious beliefs and social customs are very unique to this country. Fire is considered sacred and worshipped - it also is a part of all celebrations.

More than 75% of the population live in rural areas and below the poverty line. Approximately 200,000 people sustain burn injury yearly and about 100,000 die. This high incidence is largely due to illiteracy, poor living conditions, floor level cooking, poverty, traditional loose garments, and stressful life.

Females between 18-30 years suffer more than males. Approximately 80% of burns are suicidal due to marital problems, love failure, poor socioeconomic status , torture by in-laws over failure to produce children especially sons as daughters are under valued and seen as a liability. The commonest homicidal burns is due to bride burning by dissatisfied in-laws due to dowry demands. Young girls sustain chemical burns when they reject advances by the local hoodlums.

Children sustain burns due to negligence, overcrowding due to joint family system. Floor level cooking makes it easy for children to crawl and overturn the hot vessel. Many of them stay in one room huts with no electricity. The cat or the rat topples the kerosene lamp. Lack of supervision by adults and improper handling of fireworks. Finally children sit around open fire to warm themselves during winter seasons.

Men usually sustain electrical injuries largely due to illegal connections with exposed wires, or stepping on a live wire hanging loose on the ground in the field. They also sustain chemical burns when used as weapons of assault in domestic disputes, jealousy.

Although burns is a major problem in India . It has not received the attention it deserves probably due to the cost which imposes a severe burden on the limited resources. The government health system is unable to keep pace with the population explosion, further pushing down burn care to a much lower slot than it deserves. Lack of adequate burn centers, delay in transportation and initiation of treatment, prohibitive cost of treatment, and lack of financial resources adds to the grim scenario. In addition shortage of blood in the blood bank due to government policy to stop blood donation camps, and the current law in India not allowing use of cadaver skin. The dearth of skin substitutes due to its cost , have all hampered a total early excision. To add to this problem the potential risk of AIDS transmission has restricted the use of amnion as a cost effective skin cover.

Further the problem is compounded by the colored Indian skin which is more prone to hypertrophic scarring and keloid formation, non availability of pressure garments, in most centers , and even if it is available the general compliance is poor because of hot and humid climate -summer starts from february -october with temperatures ranging from 40-50 degree C with 75-90 % humidity.

Despite the severity of problems and short comings we have discovered not only limitations but also wonders of treatment. The concept of cost effective approach has enabled us to save many lives, shorten hospital stay, cut expenses and still maintain quality care . Strategies adapted to suit the limited resources.

Tips to Improve Burn Care in Developing Countries

1. Probably the significant progress has been the understanding of the concept of burn team.
2. Resuscitation-since all formulas adequately resuscitate patients we use Brooks formula with 5% D/S which costs rupees 17 when compared to RL 32 rupees.
3. Support of hypermetabolic response -continuous enteral feeding to maintain the calorie intake by using simple food , prepared in the hospital dietary dept which is acceptable and economical

1500 ml contains 1514 calories with 58 gms of protein and costs rupees 30.

4. Local wound care:
   - If the wound is 2nd degree superficial burns, amnion is used as skin cover.
   - If 3rd degree than 10-20% excised at a given time -bleeding is reduced by using monopolar/bipolar cautery, tournique, adrenal packs.
   - **Control of infection:** Frequent use of biopsies to guide administration of systemic antimicrobials is carried out by FNAC to detect and evaluate the progression of burn wound colonization. This is simple, easy, and painless method, yet sensitive and specific for bacterial quantitation for detection of sepsis.

     MRSA infection: Universal precaution like isolation, repeated hand washing with soap and water followed by spirit wash. Daily cleaning of burn rooms and furnitures with soap and water 7%. Lysol and linen washed with dakins Treatment-nasal carriers -2% mupirocin. Local wound infection-daily dressing with dakins or betadine.

     Systemic sepsis: Teicoplanin and vancomycin followed by rifampicin and septran for 2 weeks.

5. Management of sepsis:
   - The first clinical sign of sepsis is a rise in respiratory rate, at this stage ABG is done to treat the PO_2. If low try 40-60% venturi. If it still does not come up then use CPAP assembled at CMC -Vellore (10,000 rupees -$250). This abviates the need for endotracheal intubation.
   - Post operative skin care is by simple cost effective easily available in all houses coconut oil which is traditionally used in all houses no matter how poor the family background is:
     - Pressure garment -Ace wrap cotton is used for pressure.

Problems to be solved:

- Financial resources
- Provide adequate burn centers
- Educate the public

- Control population explosion
- Provide infrastructure.

Hurdles in Burn Prevention Strategies.

- Poor safety measures at home and work place.
- Poverty and illiteracy.

Advantages

- India has tremendous potential to do more.
- We have highly trained and skilled professionals.
- Technology is advanced and available.
- Metro cities have centers of excellence, where quality of care offered is of high level.

Challenge

- To expand our efforts in prevention and education.
- To decrease overall health care costs and make adequate funds available.
- To convince government -the importance of skin bank.

INDEX

A

B

E

F

R

U

V

W

X

Z